The Journal of the H
Management System
Volume 12, Number 2

HEALTHCARE INFORMATION MANAGEMENT®

JULIE FOREMAN, *Manager, Editorial Services*

BEENA RAO, *Copy Editor*

KATRINA YOUNG, *Editorial Assistant*

1997-1998 HIMSS PUBLICATIONS COMMITTEE

Chair
Scott A. Klink, *FHIMSS, Telecommunications Manager, Floyd Memorial Hospital, New Albany, Indiana*

Board Liaison
Pam Matthews, *FHIMSS, Senior Consultant, KPMG Peat Marwick, LLP, Atlanta, Georgia*

Publications Committee
Joseph P. Brown, *Director, Healthcare Consulting, Epic USA, Inc., Natick, MA*

Rick Caldwell, *Assistant Executive Director and CIO, Mississippi Baptist Medical Center, Jackson, Mississippi*

Beverly Clemmons, *Product Manager, ActaMed Corporation, Atlanta, GA*

James H. Ford, F*HIMSS, CHE, Senior Management Engineer, Baptist Memorial Health Care System, Memphis, Tennessee*

Joseph Shapiro, *Applications Manager, Oregon Health Sciences University, Info Technologies Group, Portland, Oregon*

Nancy G. Stetson, *RN, FHIMSS, Consultant, Kurt Salmon Associates, Atlanta, Georgia*

Julie Foreman, *Staff Liaison, Healthcare Information and Management Systems Society*

Katrina Young, *Editorial Assistant, Healthcare Information and Management Systems Society*

David Gabriel, *Editorial Assistant, Healthcare Information and Management Systems Society*

HEALTHCARE INFORMATION MANAGEMENT® (ISSN 1066–906X) is published quarterly by the Healthcare Information and Management Systems Society (HIMSS) and Jossey-Bass Publishers. Subscription to this publication is a benefit of membership in HIMSS. Statements and opinions appearing in articles and departments of the journal are those of the authors and do not necessarily reflect the position of HIMSS.

COPYRIGHT © 1998 by the Healthcare Information and Management Systems Society and Jossey-Bass Inc., Publishers.

All rights reserved. No part of this publication may be reproduced, stored in a retrieval system, or transmitted, in any form or by any means, electronic, mechanical, photocopying, recording or otherwise, without the prior written permission of Jossey-Bass Inc., Publishers, 350 Sansome Street, San Francisco, CA 94104-1342.

"HIMSS," "Healthcare Information and Management Systems Society," "Healthcare Information Management," and the HIMSS symbol are registered trademarks.

Note: Starting with Volume 10, Number 1, each volume of *Healthcare Information Management*® begins with the Spring issue. Volumes 1–9 began with the Winter issue.

Healthcare Information Management® is indexed by the American Hospital Association's Hospital Literature Index and HEALTH, a joint database of the AHA and the National Library of Medicine.

TO ORDER subscriptions, single issues, or article reprints, please refer to the Ordering Information page at the back of this issue.

ADDRESS CHANGES: *Postmaster:* Send to Jossey-Bass Publishers, 350 Sansome Street, San Francisco, CA 94104-1342. *HIMSS subscribers:* Send to Healthcare Information and Management Systems Society, 230 East Ohio Street, Suite 500, Chicago, IL 60611-3201. *Non-HIMSS subscribers:* Send to Jossey-Bass Publishers, 350 Sansome Street, San Francisco, CA 94104-1342.

Manufactured in the United States of America on Lyons Falls Turin Book. This paper is acid-free and 100 percent totally chlorine-free.

CONTENTS

EDITOR'S INTRODUCTION ... 1

ARTICLES

A Call Center Primer ... 5
William Durr

Why A Call Center? And Why Now? ... 19
Boyd K. Honeycutt, MD, MBA, FACP; Suellen Burke

Integrating Heterogeneous Healthcare Call Centers ... 29
Karen M. Peschel, LPN; William C. Reed, FHIMSS, FCHIME; Krista Salter

Managing Care Through High-Quality, Customer-Focused Service: HealthCall ... 41
Mary Ann Baxter; Pamela S. Blankenship; Edward Kornacki; Cathy McMahan; Bill Epstein

Call Centers in Healthcare: The Experience of One Health Maintenance Organization ... 53
Kathleen A. Christopherson, BSN, RN

How Technology Can Make You a Hero with Your Customers ... 59
Dick Herrmann; Mary Bryant

Creating a Vision for Your Medical Call Center ... 71
Julie L. Barr; Sue Laufenberg; Brian L. Sieckman

Developing Web-Based Knowledge Management Systems for Healthcare Call Centers ... 87
John R. Odden

Developing A Successful Call Center: One Hospital's Story ... 97
Donna M. Campbell

One Ringy Dingy: Call Centers of the Nineties ... 107
Gerard M. Nussbaum, MS, CPA, CMA, RCDD; Star P. Ault, MS, MBA

Providence Health Plan Call Center: A Case Study in Innovation and Integration ... 121
Miriam Odermann; Gregory J. Petras; Janeen Cook

Customer Service Call Center Infrastructure Redesign ... 127
Stephen Pratt; Jeffrey Johnson

HIMSS RESOURCES ... 139

CALL FOR PAPERS
Healthcare Information Management®
1999 Editorial Calendar

Spring 1999
Topic   Post-Acute Care
Proposal Deadline   July 1, 1998
Manuscript Deadline   September 15, 1998

Summer 1999
Topic   Clinical Decision Support
Proposal Deadline   October 1, 1998
Manuscript Deadline   December 15, 1998

Fall 1999
Topic   Clinical Systems Applications
Proposal Deadline   January 4, 1999
Manuscript Deadline   March 15, 1999

Summer 1999
Topic   Telehealth
Proposal Deadline   April 1, 1999
Manuscript Deadline   June 15, 1999

Prospective authors may obtain a copy of the HIMSS Writer's Guidelines by contacting HIMSS at 312/664-HIMSS (4467), Web Site: http://www.himss.org, E-mail: himss@himss.org, or Fax-on-Demand Document Service: 800/HIMSS-11 (800/446-7711) Document #.

Healthcare Information Management®
Writer's Guidelines
Healthcare Information Management ® is a quarterly journal devoted to professional development issues in healthcare information and management systems. It is published by the Healthcare Information and Management Systems Society, Chicago, IL, a not-for-profit membership organization dedicated to promoting a better understanding of healthcare information and management systems, and to the professional growth of its members.

Readership and Circulation
Healthcare Information Management ® circulation is approximately 12,000. The primary audience includes professionals in hospital administration, information systems, management engineering, telecommunications, clinical professions, consultants, university program faculty, and managers in other sectors of the healthcare field. *Healthcare Information Management* ® is indexed by the American Hospital Association's Hospital Literature Index and the National Library of Medicine's on-line bibliographic data base, *Health*.

Manuscript Submission
Healthcare Information Management ® seeks articles in the following formats:
- Market Analysis: Articles defining the state of the field, or its various components, and identifying their information and management system needs.
- Technology Overview: Articles surveying and defining the key enabling technologies and/or business methodologies for the field or its components (mobile computing, relational databases, handwriting/voice recognition, etc.), formulas for budgeting and/or needs assessment.
- Case Studies: Articles explaining who, what, when, how, and why of a particular problem or challenge, and how it was solved, or solution proposal.
- Book/Literature/Resource Review: In-depth articles reviewing a book or resource (including on-line products and services). Articles surveying a variety of resources to further readers' understanding of the field.

Authors should submit a one page proposal including the following information:
- One-to-two paragraph abstract
- Complete name, title, address, telephone number, fax number, and e-mail address of all potential authors

Send to Julie Foreman, Manager, Editorial Services, HIMSS, 230 E. Ohio St., Suite 500, Chicago, IL 60611. You will be contacted upon acceptance of the article.

Manuscript Preparation
Length
- 3,000–5,000 words, single-spaced, excluding figures, tables, and appendices.
- Author biographies are limited to 30 words and should appear at the end of text.

Layout
- Use standard sized 8–1/2 x 11" white paper with one-inch margins on all sides.
- Use single column format, single-spaced, ragged right.

Font
- Use 10 point type for body copy. Serif fonts such as Palatino or Times Roman are preferred.
- Text included in charts, graphs, and figures should be as large as possible to maximize readability.

Headings
- DO NOT include an abstract at the beginning of the paper.
- DO NOT leave blank pages or columns within the document.
- DO NOT start each new section on a new page.
- Major headings should be in CAPITAL LETTERS, 12 point, flush left within the column. Please DO NOT bold.
- Subheadings should be in upper and lowercase 10 point, flush left within the column on a separate line following paragraph. Please DO NOT bold.
- Sub-subheadings should be in upper and lower case, 10 point, flush left within the column at the beginning of the paragraph. They may be either bold or italicized to set off title from body text.

Figures/Graphs/Charts
- Limit the number of figures, graphs, and charts to three.
- Assign a title and figure number to each.
- In text, refer to all figures, graphs, and charts by title and figure number.
- Label x and y axis of every graph.
- Distinguish bars or pie chart sections by pattern, not color.
- DO NOT include graphics in the computer file version of the paper. Save all graphics in a separate text file. Use the figure title and number for file name.
- Include two hard copies of each graphic (if graphics are not retrievable they will be scanned). This is mandatory.

File Format

Required Media: Mac 3.5" 1.4mb or 800k or PC/Win 3.5" 1.4 mb

Provide text as straight text, following the minimal formatting guidelines previously stated. Save figures and graphics in a separate text file. Page breaks, **bolding**, <u>underlining</u>, *italicizing,* etc. are strongly discouraged. Save each figure and graph as a separate document. The original hard copy layout of the document will be used as a reference.

Acceptable file formats (**TEXT ONLY**):

Word Processors:

Mac	*PC*
Word	Text
Excel	RTF
Powerpoint	Word (DOS & Windows)
Photoshop	WordPerfect (Dos & Windows)
Quark	
Pagemaker	
Claris Works	

Note: If using Windows, please save in Word 6.0 or below.

Acceptable file formats (Graphics):

Mac (PICT) to PC	PC to Mac (PICT)
TIFF	PC Paintbrush.PCX
Windows Bitmap.BMP	TIFF
Windows Metafile.WMF	Windows.BMP
Windows Metafile.WMF	

Electronic Submission

Manuscripts that do not contain figures or graphs may be submitted via e-mail. Send to jforeman@himss.org.

Style and Presentation

- Use standard spelling, style, reference, and grammar guides such as *Webster's New Collegiate Dictionary, the American Medical Association Manual of Style,* and *The Elements of Style.*
- Use active sentences and be specific. Back up generalities with examples. Avoid jargon.
- All articles will be copy edited and, where necessary, rewritten. The process by which authors may review and approve changes is defined in the Letter of Agreement.

References

- Submit only complete references.
- In the text body, numbers should appear in square brackets [1]. In reference list, numbers should be in bullet format.
- Use AMA style for references. Please refer to the following examples:

Books:

1. Foreman, J.F. & Fulkerson, W.F. (1997). *HIMSS Writer's Guidelines.* Chicago, IL: Healthcare Information and Management Systems Society.

Periodicals:
2. Gabriel, D. (1996). New team, new look. *HIMSS News, 6, 12,* 10–12.
- Reference list should begin on a separate page following the document.
- References should be numbered and listed in the text body in order of appearance.

Submission Checklist
1. Manuscript on 3/5" Macintosh or PC disk following formatting guidelines.
2. One hard copy, formatted with art and figures.
3. Two (2) separate copies of each piece of art.
4. Signed letter of agreement.
5. Send to: Healthcare Information Management®
                Attention: Julie Foreman, Manager, Editorial Services
                230 E. Ohio Street, Suite 600
                Chicago, IL 60611–3201

EDITOR'S INTRODUCTION

Healthcare Call Centers: Realizing Service, Satisfaction, Revenue and Retention

As editor of this volume of *Healthcare Information Management*®, I have chosen to take an editorial approach of not spending time in this introduction pointing out the excellent work of the contributing authors. I am certain you will find the collection of papers as provocative and insightful as I have.

So, let me thank this issue's contributors and say that your papers speak for themselves. The only general observation I will make is to say that all of the articles are remarkably fresh, free of propaganda and hype. I hope that these well-crafted contributions erase any last vestiges of skepticism about call centers as the appropriate place to start providing patients with great customer service.

Successful and competitive healthcare providers are extending improved patient engagements into life-long patient relationships because it doesn't take much to realize that a satisfied patient is more likely to become a repeat patient.

The expectations of speed, reliability, and intimacy are increasingly becoming the benchmark that patients use to measure the quality of their interaction with a healthcare enterprise. Establishing an interactive experience that is characterized by an obsession for reliability, speed, and intimacy is the most significant way to effect and forge the relationships that will characterize the successful healthcare enterprise of the next century.

I recently read an article in which the author asked why the bulk of our nation's healthcare providers' executives and managers consistently check their real-world experiences at their office doors when they get to work. We never forget that we are managers when we are the patients. Unfortunately, when we become managers, we often forget what it is like to be a patient. Most call center managers may recognize themselves for just that—managers, but seeing themselves as consumer-patients with their own hectic daily routines, they too tend to forget that we live in a world based on intimate relationships.

What we healthcare delivery professionals often fail to realize is that we now compete with better service from places we never suspected. We now compete with the likes of Citibank, Disney, and Fox and our patients are part of a world where the expectations about www.com are now the same as those of an 800 number. The line between what has been the patient-doctor relationship and the customer-company relationship is moving, blurring, and changing in different directions all at once. Increasingly, you must look further and further outside your own business segments to discover where expectations about service are being created. The identification of trends that cause patient disatisfaction can help the provider quickly adapt to changing patient preferences and tolerances.

Patients, like all customers, are part of the shift from transactional efficiencies to technical intimacies. It is the quality of the contact, not the quality of the content, that matters. There is a subtle, but sublime, understanding that patients have no way of knowing your expertise; they do know the quality of the contact. We now know empirically that the greater the quality of contact, the greater the retention. Small movements in patient retention can equate to large shifts in revenues. In fact, a small change in only a few data percentage points in patient retention can equal millions of dollars to the enterprise.

In this journal, Boyd Honeycutt, MD, MBA, points out that of patients who use a telephone to call a call center and talk with the nurse advisor, 50 to 60 percent choose self care with no visits. Another 20 to 25 percent opt for a next-day regular visit with their primary provider. Further, Dr. Honeycutt reveals that "nationwide, 80 to 85 percent of callers select self-care or next-day visits, and do not utilize emergency room or other higher intensity of site." Dr. Honeycutt also points out that satisfaction levels are high—which is important in attracting and retaining patients. It is also less expensive to retain and cultivate an existing member than it is to recruit a new one, by a factor of three or four to one. And, if the use of nurse triage programs can decrease office visits by 15 percent, then it is true that more members can be served with no addition of staff, he concludes. In the end, the numbers speak for themselves.

Time has become the most precious resource in the patient's life—isn't it in yours? We are entering a millennial generation where your customer is a patient who increasingly exploits the efficiencies of new technology. Missed connections (ringing, then a busy signal), broken transfers and improperly handled patient requirements can put reliability expectations seriously at risk and can certainly cost the healthcare enterprise much more to repair than doing it right the first time. Too much technology can turn patients off. Systems that offer functions that users don't really want and lack qualities they find important can frustrate them. Take Integrated Voice Response as an example, where there are issues about the efficiencies of long menus versus the anger of patients stuck in them (or even worse, voice mail jail). This generates a suspicion of evasive antagonism.

Patients now live in a world where their banks rarely lose their account numbers from department to department; why can't we in healthcare provide this? Patients have become so used to technology in general that they are now impatient if an agent doesn't know everything about their contacts, engagements, touches, and transactions as soon as the agent answers the phone. Patients, as consumers, do not want to waste time—you must have something meaningful to say. If you ask them they will tell you, "Stop querying me, your loyal patient, for who I am, or how I plan to pay or will pay for the plan. Chances are you already have asked me. The savings in both of our time will be enormous."The fact is, if you keep your patients waiting, you don't keep your patients. However, be leery of the misnomer of speed. If you do it fast but you don't do it right, you have sped up nothing. Focusing on transactional efficiencies over patient intimacies is a slippery slope and achieving transactional speed requires reliability of system. The call center has emerged as an environment where downtime is an emergency; an environment where the worst thing that can happen is when your patients and customers cannot reach you at all.

Call centers are, without question, at the heartbeat of today's consumer-focused healthcare enterprise. The call center is as close as you can get to your patients' vital signs without having them come in, or even more costly, go to the emergency room. The three or five minutes that a patient is engaged with your healthcare enterprise represents a "moment of truth"; and in that moment, if your patient's needs are not met expeditiously and professionally, you stand to sacrifice quality in your relationship.

Reliability, speed, and intimacy are increasingly being measured, not by the number of calls answered, but by the quality of the interactions. As a result, many call centers are beginning to see performance measured against more strategic, enterprise-wide elements, such as patient retention, satisfaction, consistency in service level, application of best business practices and, ultimately, revenue growth.

One of the industry's challenges is recognizing that vital information is often found accumulated in silos, legacy systems, and private tyrannical department domains. And, to make matters worse, much of this data may be corrupt, inaccurate, incomplete, or stored in incompatible formats or media. In addition, the typical healthcare enterprise is suffering from the sometimes dramatic inefficiencies in the current ways of integrating different patient touch-points—the chief one being the telephone.

Healthcare information management is a doubled-edged sword as new, serious issues have yet to be resolved about the privacy and handling of patient data. The unique concerns and requirements of the healthcare industry are at the forefront of candidly exploring the sensitivities around issues such as patient privacy and the Millennium Bug (Y2K) problem. Healthcare, by its very nature, is where the profound extremes of technology can be viewed as either invasive or intimate. The potential abuses and liabilities are enormous.

The most difficult challenge remains the one of attitudes—all the way up your respective corporate food chain. At some point in every major information technology and call center initiative, there is the inevitable barrier of the political turf war. Many CTI and call center projects have come to a slow, grinding halt because too many executives start ducking out of on-track meetings. Lasting and impactful healthcare revolutions have always occurred from the top down. As an Ethiopian proverb says, remember that change cannot come about when the camels at the back of the caravan get the beatings while the ones at the front hold everything up.

In today's hyper-competitive world, one in which your enterprises engage with patients through a variety of media, keeping patients loyal will demand heightened attention and greater focus from operational managers on strategic business rules, rather than the traditional efficiency measurements.

The power of information that is generated from the touch-points of a call center now makes it possible for every healthcare enterprise to remember each patient as readily as the patient can remember you. If you can't do this, then by the time you get the message from your patients, they will be long gone. That message is very clear.

When I survey the healthcare industry landscape and the efficiencies of CTI and call centers, I see many not taking advantage of the benefits. The attractiveness of call centers is:

Ability to lower cost without lowering of quality or access
Patient satisfaction
Member attraction and retention
Revenue growth
Market differentiation
Higher fees for superior service
Decreased variation across the system

The future of the competitive and successful healthcare enterprise is not only the struggle for obtaining and exploiting information, but also the cultivation of life-long patient relationships. The successful healthcare enterprise will adapt to the new paradigm of business drivers—the patients and their time. What technology is providing, be it through the telephone, Internet or skills-based routing, is more time for people to have contact with the people that they want to have contact with, while eliminating unimportant, merely frictional encounters.

We have to look at patient care from a new, different perspective—theirs. Loyal patients today know that the end-game is not about data points, it's about touch-points, and they are no longer willing to put up with unnecessary lines or queues, filling out gratuitous forms or telling telemarketers whether they have had a nice day or not. Hardware stores and credit card companies often do a better job of creating intimate customer relationship expectations than many healthcare providers do.

Up-trending relies on personalizing each patient's transactions and dialogue to improve retention and profitability. It is in the healthcare call center where service, satisfaction, revenue, and retention are realized and here are 12 excellent papers to explain exactly why.

TONI BAYCH, FHIMSS
PRINCIPAL, BAYCH::NELSON

ARTICLES

A Call Center Primer

William Durr

Overview

The first modern call center was created in a joint venture between Rockwell International Corporation and Continental Airlines 25 years ago. In the intervening years, call centers have undergone significant technological change and have been integrated into nearly every industry in industrialized countries around the world. A call center is generally defined as a "place where callers can quickly and efficiently conduct transactions with trained, skilled company representatives or obtain needed information from automated sources."

Businesses have embraced call centers for various reasons. In the beginning, call centers were used almost exclusively to generate revenue. It is therefore not surprising that airlines were the first users of call centers. They were interested in selling airplane seats, a highly perishable commodity, as efficiently as possible. After the door shuts, the empty seat represents a cost burden. So it made good sense to make it very easy for people to get through to airline agents to purchase seats.

In the past decade, call centers have assumed a bigger role in the delivery of customer service. Business executives in many industries began to recognize that competitive differentiators were difficult to sustain. Progressive firms discovered that if product differences were difficult or impossible to create, competitive advantage could be gained by making it very easy for customers to conduct business transactions with them. Call centers and the applications they serve are being established in ever-increasing numbers, and existing centers are being expanded in size and scope because they play a central role in acquiring new customers and retaining existing customers. They also accomplish these missions in the most cost-effective manner. It is for these reasons that the healthcare industry has adopted call centers for such traditional applications as claims processing and process authorization. Now call centers are being used in new applications such as nurse triage, centralized scheduling, and delivering laboratory results.

Call Center Components

Call centers are unique combinations of technology and people. Historically the people are referred to as "agents" (the influence of the airline origins); however, the terms "customer service representative" or "telephone service representative" are also gradually taking hold. The technology consists of a bewildering collection of equipment with imposing acronyms like *ACD, IVR, CTI,* and *LAN*. We should consider ourselves lucky that there are only 26 letters in our alphabet or the acronym jungle might become impenetrable. We will review each major component as identified in Figure 1.1.

Automatic Call Distributor. An automatic call distributor (ACD) has two functions: processing calls (that is, moving them around) and reporting on what is happening. An ACD can be implemented on various telephone switching systems such as private branch exchanges (PBX), key systems, central office (sometimes referred to as "centrex"), or on specialized platforms such as the Rockwell Spectrum. All these platforms share common elements. Telephone trunks (lines, circuits) are connected to the ACD's telephone line interface cards. Agents are connected to the ACD with either a specialized telephone instrument or with a personal computer on which a special "software telephone" program resides. A voice messaging subsystem provides announcements, information messages, and caller prompts with prerecorded phonemes, words, phrases, and sentences.

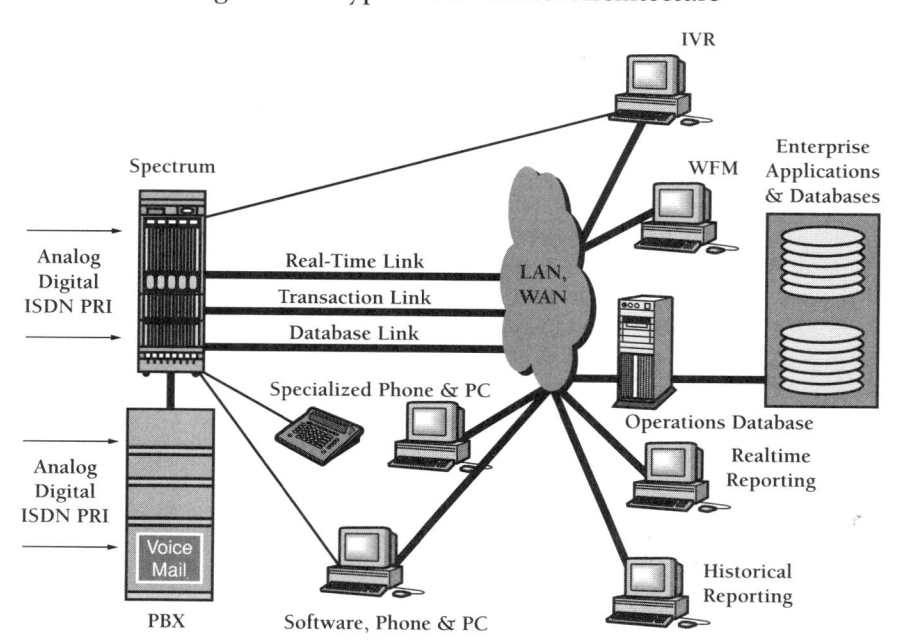

Figure 1.1. Typical Call Center Architecture

ACD systems typically have data links that connect the ACD control processor to the local are networks (LANs) and wide area networks (WANs) so prevalent in today's business enterprises. These data links enable other call center hardware/software systems to be integrated with the ACD.

Call Processing. One of the two most important functions of an ACD is to route calls. In general terms, a call route is established for each kind of transaction expected to be handled. In the routing table, the ACD is told how to deal with the caller. The ACD empowers the call center user to create his or her own, unique call processing rules within the confines of each vendor's unique routing control tools. Differences among switch vendors can be measured in tangible ways such as the number of permitted routes, the number of permitted steps in a route, how quickly changes can be made in routes, how quickly the changes take effect, and the depth of control offered.

A basic call processing route might be constructed as follows:

1. Agent group 1
2. Hold 18 seconds
3. Announcement 5
4. Music source 2
5. Hold 45 seconds
6. Announcement 10
7. Go to step 5

Callers entering this routing table would be offered to the group 1 agent who has been available the longest time. If an agent is immediately available, the caller will be immediately connected to that agent. If no agent is currently available, the caller will hear ringing for 18 seconds. This is about 3 ring cycles. During the ringing and all subsequent steps, the ACD is always looking for an available agent in group 1 and if it finds one it immediately connects the caller. After 18 seconds, the caller is connected to the announcement contained in location 5. This might be the first delay announcement or other appropriate initial message. Then the caller is connected to music source 2, which is playing an appropriate musical program. The caller will listen to this music for an additional 45 seconds before being connected to announcement 10. The loop-back step is designed to cycle callers through an endless loop of announcement location 10 every 45 seconds until the caller is connected to an available agent in group 1 or the caller abandons the attempt.

More interesting call processing capabilities are created when call center users begin to use conditional commands. In our basic call processing route example, we could have substituted a conditional statement for the first command, as shown below:

1. If more than 10 callers in queue for agent group 1, then send busy signal
2. Agent group 1

3. Hold 18 seconds
4. Announcement 5

This command relieves the call center manager from having to continually monitor conditions by predefining certain conditions and the actions to be taken when those conditions occur. In our example, the call center manager has decided that when there are 10 callers in queue for the agents in group 1, the system should send busy signals to new callers until the queue has fewer than 10 callers. Conditional routing is only as powerful as the number of conditions that can be tested. A set of useful conditions would include:

Time of day
Number of agents available
Number of agents staffed
Percentage of available agents
Number of calls waiting
Age of oldest queued call
Application service level
Application average speed of answer

The usual practice is that if the condition is met, the call processor will perform the action specified in the second part of the command. If the condition is not met the call processor will move to the next step in the table.

An example of more complex routing is as follows:

1. If number of calls waiting for agent group 11 is more than 12, then send busy signal
2. Agent group 11
3. Hold 18 seconds
4. If time of day is later than 1200, then play announcement 24 ("Good Afternoon . . ."), else play announcement 23 ("Good Morning . . .")
5. Hold 15 seconds
6. Agent group 17
7. Play announcement 22 ("Sorry for delay . . .")
8. If time of day is later than 1600 or number of messages waiting for agent group 11 is more than 15, then go to step 10, else play announcement 14 ("Apologize for delay, press 9 to leave message . . .")
9. Collect one digit from caller; if "9" go to step 15, else go to step 13
10. Play announcement 27 ("Thank you for continuing to hold")
11. Queue 45 seconds
12. Go to step 10
13. Play announcement 30 ("Sorry you're having difficulty . . .")
14. Go to step 10
15. Play announcement 15 ("Key in phone number . . .")

16. Collect 7 digits from caller; if "time-out," go to step 23
17. Play announcement 17 ("The number you entered is . . .")
18. Play digits received
19. Play announcement 18 ("If number correct press '1'")
20. Collect 1 digit from caller; if "1" go to step 21 else go to step 15
21. Play announcement 19 ("Leave message at tone")
22. End table
23. Play announcement 21 ("Did not receive phone number")
24. Play announcement 10 ("Please hold")
25. Raise priority to 6
26. Queue 999 seconds

This example illustrates how custom call processing treatments can be created. The call center manager has decided to reject new callers if the number of calls waiting for agent group 11 exceeds 12. If the number of calls waiting is less than 12, then the caller is offered to any agent in group 11. If no agents are available the caller will hear central office ringing for 18 seconds. The manager uses time of day testing to play the appropriate first delay announcement and then expands the search for an available agent to include agents in group 17. After holding for 30 seconds longer the manager has programmed the call processor to test for either 4 PM or the number of existing voice mail messages for group 11. If either condition is met, then the caller is placed in a loop in which a periodic message is played until the caller is handled or abandons. If neither condition is met, the manager has established a message-taking routine that includes capturing the caller's phone number for automatic dialing. The ability to create powerful, automatic call processing flows is usually limited only by the imagination and creativity of the call center user.

Management Information. Many experts believe that the real value of ACD systems lies in the data that the machines capture and store. The user is provided a stunning, even overwhelming, array of data including:

- Telephone circuits: Calls offered, handled, and abandoned by trunk; average connect time by trunk; trunk group all busy time; individual trunk statistics; out of service time by trunk
- Application or transaction type: Average speed of answer; service level; calls offered, handled, abandoned; average talk time; average after-call work time; average number of staffed positions; average time to abandon
- Agent performance information: Sign-on time; ACD calls handled; non-ACD calls handled; out-calls placed; average talk time; average after-call work time; average unavailable time

The user can typically either obtain such data in real-time or can ask for printed reports of different historical perspectives. Many systems now support historical records that reach back more than 1 year. Why are all these data needed?

The Role of Performance Data in the Call Center. Consider managing a grocery store. Apart from all the details connected with putting merchandise on the shelves, there is the management task connected with checking out the customers' carts. One has to worry about lengthy lines, not enough checkers, and schedules for breaks and lunches. The analogy between the grocery checkout area and a call center is really rather close. The checkers play a role exactly like that of agents while customers wait in line or queues.

There is one difference, however, between a checkout manager and a call center manager. The grocery store is a physical store while the call center is an electronic one. In the physical store, management can use all its senses to create dimensions of conditions, assess alternatives, and take corrective actions. In the electronic store, management is largely blind. The call center represents an invisible world in which faceless interaction takes place. Management attempts to understand similar dynamics in the call center as does the checkout manager in a grocery store, with the difference being, however, that they use data to provide their "view."

The trunk reports produced by nearly all systems provide important clues to whether there are enough trunks or too many trunks and whether they are working properly. Many organizations watch the last trunk in a hunt group closely for the amount of traffic it carries. The logic is that if the last trunk in a hunt group begins to carry increasing amounts of traffic, it is increasingly probable that some callers are getting busy signals.

Application reports are invaluable. They include data on the number of calls offered, handled, and abandoned, as well as agent performance statistics such as average talk time, average after-call work time, average available time, and average idle time and service level or average speed of answer. These data can be used to decide what the demand for access to the call center is and how well the demand is being satisfied.

Agent reports move one level deeper. They include detailed performance data on every individual agent in the center. The agents are collected into skill groups and group norms are calculated. Armed with these data, a baseline standard can be created for performance by agent group and each agent's performance can be compared with group norms. Identifying struggling agents is key to the success of any call center.

Historical reports for trunks, agent groups, and individual agents provide guidance in identifying trends and patterns in call demand or any of the other elements that influence service levels. Without such data, a manager cannot possibly get ballpark figures on staffing levels that support service level targets. Ultimately, the sophistication of call processing table construction is irrelevant if nobody is available to talk to the caller.

Voice Mail. Everyone is familiar with voice mail. In the general business world, voice mail can be simultaneously valued and reviled. In call centers, voice mail can be used to prevent callers from waiting too long. Voice mail ports can be treated as if they were an agent group; they can be used in routing tables to give callers a choice after a certain period of waiting in queue. Callers can decide for themselves if they want to remain in queue for a live agent or if they wish to leave a voice mail message and receive a call back later. This is an important tool that can help solve brief mismatches between staff and call demands.

There can also be applications for individual agent voice mailboxes, particularly in healthcare claims processing. Often any appropriately skilled agent can handle an initial claims call. But if the transaction requires subsequent calls and interactions, it is more efficient for the caller to speak with the same agent. Return calls to a particular agent will frequently find that agent already engaged. So individual agent mailboxes can be valuable. One caveat for standalone ACD systems is that they should interface with the associated PBX's voice mail system so that the call center agents do not have a voice mail system that is different from that used by the rest of the enterprise.

Interactive Voice Response. More and more people are familiar with and respond positively toward interactive voice response (IVR) systems. The attraction is easy to understand. IVR systems transform an ordinary Touch-Tone telephone into a computer terminal of sorts. An IVR is a multimedia personal computer system. It stores a prerecorded voice in phonemes, words, phrases, and entire statements. In addition, IVR systems have access to computer databases. The caller interacts with the IVR by listening to prerecorded prompt messages and responding by depressing Touch-Tone keys, by speaking digits, or by responding "yes" or "no." The IVR system uses the caller inputs to retrieve data from the database and verbalize information of interest to the caller.

Using this technology, simple transactions can be completed without human agent involvement. Because computers are tireless, IVR applications are available to callers 24 hours a day, 365 days a year. The kinds of applications that can be successfully conducted via IVR technology are unlimited. In general, if a caller can be identified by a numeric account number or personal identification number and the agent uses that number to access a computer screen to read data back to the caller, then that application probably can be automated by IVR technology. This frees agents to deal with more complex transactions.

A specialized IVR application in most call centers is known as "auto attendant." In the auto attendant application, the caller is greeted by an IVR system and then prompted to key in "1" for this, "2" for that, "3" for another thing, and so on. The caller's digit-responses are used to direct the call to the most appropriately skilled agent group. Another generalized auto attendant application involves prompting the caller to enter a unique personal identification. The caller's identification is sent by the IVR system to a computer telephony integration (CTI) server so that specific information relating to that caller appears on the agent's screen as the caller is connected to that agent.

Computer Telephony Integration. CTI is a happy marriage between voice systems and business data processing systems. Before CTI, the only connecting point between the ACD and the computer system driving the agent terminals was the agent. The agent reacted to data supplied by the ACD system and used the data processing system to handle the transaction request. For example, the ACD system can inform the agent via the agent's instrument of the number that the caller dialed, thereby identifying the kind of transaction the caller wishes to conduct. Still the agent must work the computer keyboard to bring up the appropriate transaction screen.

With CTI and appropriate software running on the host side, the ACD system can pass the number dialed and the position number of the agent to whom the caller will be connected. The computer system software can use that information to automatically display the correct transaction type screen on the correct agent display. This saves precious seconds for each transaction. We know that seconds saved in a transaction have dramatic positive operational results.

Beyond this is the almost magical application involving the combination of automatic number identification and CTI. First the ACD receives the calling party's telephone number from the network or prompts the caller to enter in a unique identification number. The ACD sends this information and the agent position that will handle the caller. The computer system can use the originating telephone number or unique identification number as an access key into the customer database. Then the computer can display customer data on the screen in front of the agent as the caller's voice enters the agent's ear. Knowing who is calling before answering the telephone facilitates big time savings.

Workforce Management Software Packages. About 25 percent of existing call centers make use of workforce management software packages (variously referred to WFM or forecasting, staffing, and scheduling). It is surprising that more call centers do not make use of these software packages. WFM systems are available in a broad range of capabilities and sophistication. Usually these software packages deal with forecasting call volumes based on historical data, calculating staff required for a desired service level goal, taking into account individual agent preferences for work patterns and days off, and creating a set of individual schedules. This kind of software attempts to minimize the labor involved in providing an optimal service level.

WFM software packages tend to be organized along similar lines. The system usually collects data from an ACD by interfacing with a printer port or directly accessing the ACD performance database. As the software package collects data, it builds a model of that call center's operating environment. The software database captures all the myriad patterns experienced by call centers. Call arrival patterns emerge based on time, day, date, and month. Armed with this historical data and cognizant of all the patterns, WFM software is capable of producing call volume forecasts with amazing precision.

The complexity of these software systems largely depends on work rules and agent preferences. The user defines what kinds of work patterns exist. There are many permutations and combinations of total shift length, number of breaks, length of breaks, meal breaks, and so on. Definition of work patterns involves deciding when permissible start times shall occur, how long after the start time the first break should be scheduled, how long the agent should work after the last break before ending the shift, and so on.

The end result is a set of individual agent schedules that attempts to cover the call volume while satisfying agent requirements. But this is not the end of the software's functionality. Having planned for the forthcoming week, that week must actually be experienced. Schedule management is an important task in this regard. Inevitably, agents will call in sick, have car trouble, and require time off for numerous reasons. These exceptions to the planned schedule need to be entered into the system so that management can determine whether the service level goal can still be reached.

In a similar fashion, WFM systems provide call center management with important capabilities in regard to future planning. For example, training is an on-going activity in most call centers. The problem has always been to schedule training so that it does not have a negative impact on service level. By entering training into the WFM system as a future exception, the software can reserve agent time for important training and still ensure proper coverage.

Costs and Benefits

For someone new to the industry, this appears to be a formidable technological array with enormous costs. Can it be justified? Consider the typical call center cost breakdown depicted in Figure 1.2.

In most call centers that use toll-free ("800") numbers, the relative cost relationship depicted is fairly accurate. The overwhelming cost is that of labor. Fully burdened labor can easily cost a firm $50,000 annually for one moderately skilled and moderately paid agent. While the cost of transmission continues to decrease, in most call centers it represents the next biggest expense.

Figure 1.2. Typical Five–Year Call Center Cost Elements

Technology Cost - 10%
Transmission Cost - 25%
Labor Cost 65%

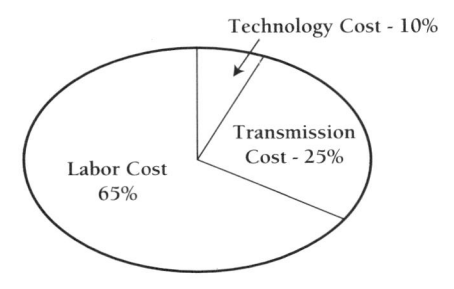

Typical 5 Year Call Center Cost Elements

Call center technology rarely exceeds 10 percent of the total cost of the operation, and this percentage also includes data processing expenses.

What are some typical benchmark prices for call center technology? ACD systems are frequently discussed in terms of price per agent seat. Powerful ACD systems can be purchased for about $3500 per seat. IVR systems are usually discussed in terms of price per port (where a port is a telephone circuit pathway into the system). Typical prices for IVR technology are about $1500 per port. Voice mail is not usually priced separately and is generally included in the ACD costs. The cost of WFM software is highly variable depending on the range of feature options. Plan on spending $50,000 to $80,000 for each site. Lastly, CTI costs are very difficult to bracket. CTI projects frequently involve the acquisition of some standard components and customization efforts. It is not unusual for CTI projects to start at $100,000 and escalate upward to seven figures.

So with all this expense how can the costs be justified? The technology is used as a lever against the two large costs of labor and transmission. The Greek mathematician Archimedes is believed to have said that if he was given a lever big enough and a place to stand, he could move the earth. So it is for the call center manager. The tools, costly though they may be perceived to be, provide the lever and the place to stand so that the knowledgeable call center manager can control the costs.

Issues and Problems

The concerns of call center managers and supervisors can easily be listed. In various seminars, identification of these concerns leads to heads nodding in agreement. A good generic list of issues and problems would include the following:

1. Agent attrition rate is too high
2. Motivation: New hires, old timers
3. How to balance staff-to-call load
4. How to deal with surges in average speed of answer
5. Which metric should I manage?
6. How to provide coverage during breaks and lunches
7. How to keep agents on the phone
8. How to properly evaluate agent performance
9. How to measure and manage quality
10. How to provide better, more cost-effective training
11. How to calculate cost per call and minimize it
12. How to get real value from all those ACD reports

This list is interesting for several reasons. One, most of the items relate to call center managers wanting to know how to accomplish a particular task. The problems are known; it is the workable solutions that elude us. Second, most of the issues and problems deal with people not technology. This means that technology's role is understood and used appropriately for the most part. Making the mix of technology and people work efficiently appears to be among the problems.

Call centers are difficult to run successfully because of the following observations.

- Call centers are unique blends of people and technology.
- Many variables affect performance.
- One only controls a few of them.
- The variables are constantly changing.

One of the special problems facing healthcare call centers is a tendency to create many smaller agent groups. This is somewhat marketing-initiated; it is also due to the specialized training and myriad options and differences that abound in healthcare contracts. The net result is that small agent teams are dedicated to handling calls from a given customer population. One of the ironies of call center operations is that small agent groups are notoriously difficult to manage for consistent good service levels. It is not until an agent group grows to be about 50 agents that large team economies begin to be realized.

Future Trends in the Call Center

Over the next 5 years, call center operations and technology will be altered by two dominant trends. The first is the Internet and the second is what can be termed the "balkanization" of technology.

The Internet and the Call Center. The Internet is washing across industrialized societies and promises to exact changes not unlike those effected by the printing press and mass production technologies. While the Internet is today mostly a vast electronic library, its future promise lies in its ability to become the next dominant communications appliance in combination with low-cost yet powerful multimedia personal computers. Already individuals and organizations are experimenting with voice over the World Wide Web. The Internet is a useful, already widely deployed protocol that is capable of handing voice, textual data, and images. The Internet will only get better at transporting multimedia and mixed media transactions.

I recall watching old Flash Gordon serial episodes as a child. Among many fascinating technologies, I found the video/phone to be the most interesting. I could not wait until science and industry brought a communication device into the market that would permit people to see and speak to each other in real time. Well, it is almost here. In addition to speaking and seeing each other, people can send each other data files and graphics.

This promises to utterly transform electronic commerce. Call centers have been attempting to replace direct human interaction with a brand of remote, faceless interaction. To be successfully implemented it requires special training, effort, and extra time. Humans are visual creatures after all. Reintroducing the visual element into call center transactions will absolutely change the nature of the remote interaction for the best. We will have come nearly full circle and return to a more humane, albeit still remote, interaction that is also natural and highly personal.

The Balkanization of ACD Systems. The second change deals with how the call center technology itself is changing over time. In the beginning, ACD systems were totally proprietary and self-contained. They scanned trunk and agent ports for state changes in real-time. They processed calls according to user rules. They generated operations information and delivered it in real-time to supervisor screens and printed historical reports. Just as the Balkan region of Europe splintered into ethnic nations earlier this century, the ACD has undergone some splintering of its own.

The first change is related to the ACD database. Instead of being internal and closed, most ACD systems provide for a standard database provisioned on a LAN server. While the vendor offers data retrieval tools as part of the product, the user is free to use existing information systems tools such as PowerBuilder, Visual Basic, and even Excel.

The next component to splinter off the ACD and on to the increasingly ubiquitous LAN/WAN computing environment is the agent telephone instrument. Most fully featured ACD systems have a proprietary agent telephone instrument. They typically have large special function keys and displays to simplify and increase call handling speed. Recently, several leading vendors introduced software suites that eliminate the physical telephone instrument. The software places a phone panel or toolbar on the personal computer screen while the agent's application runs as normal. When the phone panel software is Telephone Application Program Interface–compliant (TAPI, a standard promoted by Microsoft Corporation for integrating personal computers and telephone operations), interesting first party CTI applications can be developed inexpensively and quickly.

A third emerging area of change is control over call processing itself. When first introduced, ACD call processing commands were relatively crude and simplistic. Later, call processing was improved with the concepts of conditional commands. More recently, call processing practices were again improved with the concepts often referred to as "skill-based routing." The common element among this progression of capabilities is that the ACD is always referencing itself. Outbound telemarketing and database routing require a different approach. In outbound telemarketing campaigns, specialized software outside the ACD takes control of the switching and call processing logic and tells the ACD what to do step by step: what numbers to dial, at what pace, which agent gets connected to a live answer, etc. In database routing, leading-edge companies have decided to process calls in relation to the value of the caller to the firm. Good customers get good service, and average customers get average service. The value of a customer to a firm is likely to be in enterprise databases, which cannot be summarized inside an ACD routing table. So third party software is being created, which works in lockstep with ACD systems. The caller's identity is determined by the ACD and sent to the third party database routing software module, which determines the value of the caller and assembles a history of the relationship. The module tells the ACD what to do with this particular caller and coordinates the delivery of the screens to the agent eventually connected to the caller. What we see unfolding is the disassociation of the switch control processes from the switching engine itself.

Summary

Call centers are strategically and tactically important to many industries, including the healthcare industry. Call centers play a key role in acquiring and retaining customers. The ability to deliver high-quality and timely customer service without much expense is the basis for the proliferation and expansion of call centers. Call centers are unique blends of people and technology, where performance indicates combining appropriate technology tools with sound management practices built on key operational data. While the technology is fascinating, the people working in call centers and the skill of the management team ultimately make a difference to their companies.

About the Author

William Durr is a Senior Manager with Rockwell Electronic Commerce Division.

Why A Call Center? And Why Now?

Boyd K. Honeycutt, MD, MBA, FACP; Suellen Burke

Over a dozen years ago, in the mid–1980s, one of my patients asked a question that turned out to be a real eye-opener for me. He said, "Sometimes I don't know whether I need to come to see you or not. I hate to waste your time and my time with things that a little advice could take care of over the phone. Why don't you put one of your more experienced nurses, one that has been around long enough to know how to talk to people, on a phone to just answer questions and give advice?" My first reaction was to list all the reasons why that would not work. Doctors were trained to see their patients, and taught that it was not possible to really practice "good" medicine over the phone. Later, as I reflected on his comments, I began to wonder if he hadn't hit on something that could satisfy patients, make the physician's life easier at times, and actually help lower the cost of care. Then I discovered that there were other people who had already thought of this and had been doing it successfully for years.[1,2] Of course, it was not called "demand management" back then! As technology has advanced over the past decade or so, opportunities for expansion of services provided by a call center have increased enormously. Now the ability to integrate telephonic technology with electronic technology has further expanded capabilities.

Background

The growth of managed care and the trend toward capitation as the predominant method of reimbursement to providers has driven much of the interest in call centers and the various functions performed by them.[3] Due to the pressure on managed care organizations (MCOs) to lower prices for purchasers, MCOs have developed strategies to provide appropriate care at a lower cost. A complete listing and analysis of those strategies is beyond the scope of this article, but among the most common are use of midlevel providers, disease management programs, and demand management initiatives. For the purposes of this article, demand management is defined as "a process that seeks to control access by matching patient needs with the most cost-efficient kind of service and site of service possible, while encouraging patient participation in the process with a long-term goal of patient learning and self care."[4,5] It is important to emphatically state here that demand management is not a method to deny care but rather a way to help patients make informed decisions to lead to the outcome stated, that is, most appropriate care at the most cost-efficient site. There may be incentives for patients (or providers) to encourage acceptance of, and cooperation with, demand management policies, such as differential copayments and coinsurance.

The primary focus of this article will be the call center, which I refer to as a front-end intervention in the overall demand management strategy. The term "front end" is used to indicate that the intervention should occur early in the patient's decision-making process. It should be available when the patient is deciding whether to seek care, what kind of care, and where. Although the terms "nurse triage" and "nurse call center" are used interchangeably, they really include more than nurse triage. Triage is probably a poor term for this work, which might better be called nurse decision support or nurse-guided care choices. That is really what it is about—giving the patients the information and the "empowerment" to make better decisions about where and when to seek care.

It has been well chronicled over the past couple of decades that there is tremendous unexplained variation in physicians' practices and the provision of care. Studies have repeatedly documented that 40 percent to 50 percent of visits to emergency departments are not necessary, and could have been handled in a less acute setting. Similarly, studies have shown that 30 percent to 40 percent of visits to primary care physicians' offices are inappropriate and could have been postponed or handled over the telephone. One conclusion from these studies is that people often do not know how or when to use the healthcare system, as my patient stated few years ago. This uncertainty over how and when to use the healthcare system results in overutilization and increased costs. To illustrate, assume that a health maintenance organization (HMO) has to pay out $250 every time a patient visits an emergency room, and an HMO with 100,000 members has roughly 9000 emergency room encounters per year. If one half of those were eliminated, the HMO would save over one million dollars, which could be used for other more appropriate or necessary services. If the providers in this HMO had to pay a capitation fee and took full financial risk for these visits, they would save the dollars. This ability to save money, regardless of who gets the savings, is one of the attractions of a demand management service, or more specifically, the nurse-directed care aspect of a call center as a component of demand management.

Today's patients are generally well educated and informed. They have access to an incredible array of information sources like the daily newspapers, television, and the Internet. However, their information is often incomplete or one-sided and expert help may be required to make sense of the confusing and occasionally conflicting mass of information. Patients and their families want information and help, and they want it available to them at a time and place of their choice. MCOs with call centers that provide 24–hour service with nurses advising patients and with access to menu-driven programs where patients can learn about specific conditions have a competitive advantage in the market. Further, if a patient can make one call and get sound advice regarding a medical question or condition, receive accurate information about benefits, and schedule an appointment with the appropriate provider, he or she will be a satisfied patient. If that can be accomplished with little time spent on hold and no unnecessary "hand-offs" from one operator to another, the satisfaction will be even higher.

Indications are that 50 percent to 60 percent of patients who call a center and talk with the nurse advisor choose self care with no visit. Another 20 percent to 25 percent opt for a next-day regular office visit with their primary provider. Nationwide, some 80 percent to 85 percent of callers select self care or next-day visits, and do not use the emergency room or other high-intensity site of service. When patient satisfaction surveys include these patients, the satisfaction levels are high—usually over 90 percent are satisfied or very satisfied with the advice received.[6,7] Some patients even stay with a particular MCO because of the availability of advice and the apparent caring attitude of the nurse advisors. This satisfaction rating is important in attracting and retaining patients. Attracting patients means growth and increased revenue, while retaining patients helps with growth and contributes to the stability of a plan. It is less expensive to retain a member than to recruit a new one, by a factor of 3 or 4 to 1.

In the world of managed care today, one of the most important success factors is volume, that is, number of covered lives. If use of nurse triage programs can decrease office visits by 15 percent, as has been documented in some MCOs, more members can be accommodated with no addition of staff.[8] Those MCOs that can learn to manage larger patient loads with no increase in staff and no increase in bricks and mortar (equating to lower fixed costs) will have a huge competitive advantage. This is especially true in a capitation-based environment.[9] Demand management techniques provide an avenue to that end, and a call center is the centerpiece for a strong demand management program. The mergers and acquisitions prevalent in the healthcare industry today mean larger numbers of covered lives in integrated systems of care. It should be possible to gain financial savings by centralizing call center functions for the system and to decrease variation across the system. As integrated systems and MCOs try to differentiate themselves in the marketplace, a smoothly operating multifunctional call center can help with that differentiation. A call center that adds value in the ways described is viewed as desirable by the purchasers, and could potentially lead to higher premium levels for the MCO or integrated system.

These features, then, explain the attractiveness of call centers to MCOs: ability to lower costs without lowering quality and access; patient satisfaction;

member attraction and retention; revenue growth; differentiation in the marketplace; potential to support higher premiums; and decreased variation across the entire system. All these add up to significant competitive market advantage. It is difficult to find concrete figures about savings from call centers. Literature from around the country suggests that investments in call centers return between $2 and $4 for each dollar spent; however, some MCOs report higher returns while a few have been disappointed with their results.[10,11] At present, these are fairly soft numbers, but with time and experience, better financial outcome information will be available which should clarify the returns on investment from a call center.

Call centers can also be desirable for the provider side of the system. Screening of calls by trained nurses based on clinically proven algorithms decreases "trivial" or inappropriate visits. This allows the physician to either have more time to focus on patients who truly need care, which improves quality and patient satisfaction, or to see more patients and increase personal productivity and income. The call center nurses also decrease the burden of calls the physician has to handle during the work day or when on call, thus improving the physician's life. Most physicians who use a call center, when surveyed, say they are satisfied with the call center, and would not want to do without it. Many physicians use the call center for outbound follow-up calls also, which serves to enhance communication with patients and leads to improved quality of care. Again, these functions allow physicians to care for more patients without increasing office staff, to maintain or improve quality, to differentiate themselves, and to enhance their lifestyles. These things also result in increased revenues and increased patient satisfaction in most cases.

What Should a Call Center Look Like?

Certainly it will have the nurse triage or advice function, with nurses working from established and proven protocols to help patients arrive at a sound decision regarding what care is appropriate, and when and where that care will be provided. The center should also serve as an answering service, so that the patient can complete the entire transaction with one telephone call. The nurses or other personnel in the center should be able to schedule appointments with the appropriate providers. This will avoid scheduling an appointment with the patient for the next day, and then facing barriers at the physician's office. Working from established protocols and decision algorithms the call center personnel can approve many referrals, thus streamlining that often cumbersome and time-consuming process. Access should be available to digitized information regarding specific diseases or conditions, with the patient returning to a nurse for further questions or clarification after hearing the information. The call center should be able to provide basic information about the benefits and coverage of the specific plan under which the patient is insured. The ability to conduct follow-up calls for the physicians who use the center would be a benefit. These can be conducted in a "personalized" way, providing information to the patient, letting them know of the physician's interest in their well-being, and thus being a welcome adjunct to the physician's care. The center can conduct patient profiling to identify high-risk patients who need specific interventions that improve their care and decrease costs. This aspect can be integrated with a community case manager program. All these activities have to be clearly documented, a relatively easy task with today's technology. Addition of interactive voice response (IVR) technology whereby patients can access information about results of laboratory tests or other messages is a possibility. All the services must, of course, be available 24 hours a day, even if physicians' offices may perform some of them during business hours.

The call center should be linked telephonically and electronically with all the sites it services. Ideally, the clinical record, or at least part of it, would be available to the nurses doing the triage. While they may not need it often, having it available would be useful in some circumstances, potentially leading to better quality of care. This interconnectedness would allow smooth communication between the nurses and the offices and other sites, also leading to better care. Delivery systems that can do these things well, whether they are MCOs or integrated delivery systems, will enjoy a tremendous competitive advantage in the future. A strong call center, as the linchpin of a broad demand management program, is critical to the success of other necessary programs such as disease management, community case management, and population health management. The link between telephonic services and electronic data management is essential. As integrated systems expand into new markets, having a template that can be implemented quickly in the new area is beneficial.

The Patient-Doctor Interface

Patients often want only information and reassurance, not the inconvenience and cost of a trip to the emergency room or physician's office. These services help them achieve that goal. Studies show that patients are often more averse to risks than are doctors, and when fully informed, tend to choose less risky, lower-cost treatment options than those recommended by their physicians.[4] With demand management and call center services patients can be involved in the decisions and informed of the options. However, this does not imply that any of these services can be a substitute for informed consent obtained by a physician, but rather that they are complementary. This important point bears repeating here: all these strategies help the physician take care of the patient in a more efficient way. None of them replace the physician. The goal is to direct patients to the most appropriate, most cost-effective use of resources for the problem at hand. Implemented correctly, this should increase patient satisfaction, increase provider satisfaction, lower costs, maintain or improve quality, and result in a competitive market advantage. These outcomes ought to make call centers marketable to providers and purchasers, and possibly provide the care delivery system with a way to differentiate itself and capture higher revenues.

Barriers to Implementation

If all this is so, why isn't everybody doing it? There are substantial barriers to successful implementation of call centers. Some of these are obvious, some are rooted in the predictable anxiety over any change, and some are subtle. The following is by no means an exhaustive list, but covers the most common of these barriers.

Who Owns the Call Center? One of the most controversial problems is "who will do this?" A comprehensive call center such as described here performs significant medical management and is involved in aspects of the day-to-day operations of physicians' offices. Many believe this is not the function of the MCO or HMO, and therefore the provider organization should operate the call center. In theory, a truly integrated system which "owns" all the components—the HMO, the hospital, and the employed physician network—should find it an easier task. In reality, the different legal and governance structures often found in such systems and the political issues common to all organizations make this decision problematic. Many HMOs and MCOs believe that they have to engage in demand management activities to be viable and comply with various federal and state regulatory requirements, while providers believe that medical management, including demand management and call center activity, is their purview and not that of the MCO. Then there is the question of whether to develop a center in house or to outsource it. All the ramifications of the "make-versus-buy" decision come into question here, and the answer varies depending on the organization.

Resistance from Physicians. Physician resistance is sometimes a problem. While the call center should make physicians' lives easier, a few will balk at this because it represents change from the established patterns, and this change is perceived as a loss of control. Also some of the functions could be seen as intervening inappropriately in the physician-patient relationship, which does not sit well with most physicians. It takes a lot of communication with and involvement of physicians during the development process to overcome this obstacle and be certain that this is an aid to patient care, not a barrier.

Cost. Cost is a potential barrier to implementation. Setting up a call center is an expensive proposition, possibly on the order of several million dollars if starting from scratch. The center can be built incrementally over time, with various components built into annual budgets sequentially. This strategy might not be feasible for delivery systems in very competitive markets where rapid start-up is essential.

Centralized Versus Local. The question of a centralized versus geographically distributed call center function is another potential barrier. Many believe that call centers must have "local knowledge" to give patients directions to sites of service and to provide a more intimate and personalized feel to the service. Thus, while there are financial savings associated with centralizing management and computer functions, patient service, satisfaction, and provider satisfaction must not be ignored. The issues of ownership, "turf," and political concerns must also be considered, because jobs, revenue, and employee satisfaction are involved in this decision. In large part, the answer to this question may hinge on the size of the organization, its geographic extent, and its strategic direction.

Liability. Legal liability is a significant concern. Most large call centers have operated for several years without problems. However, in a few cases, adverse outcomes have resulted from advice that later turned out to be inappropriate in the particular circumstance. Legal problems can be minimized by using several proven tactics like experienced and trained nurses; carefully designed and tested protocols; frequent revision of these protocols; documentation of all patient contacts and instructions; early follow-up by call center nurses and the patients' own physicians; clear and prompt communication with the primary physician; and proper supervision of call centers by qualified physicians.[6,12]

Market Stage and Aligned Incentives. Market stage and misalignment of incentives are potential barriers. The call center strategy described here works best in a heavily capitation-based environment, in which physicians, hospitals, and HMOs all share the risk for patient care. At the earliest, this translates into a late stage 2 managed care market, and more likely a market with stage 3 dynamics.[13] If most of the market is still receiving fees for service, patient visits to the emergency room and physicians' offices represent revenue to these providers. It makes little sense, from the providers' perspective, to try to decrease those events. While the HMO or MCO may wish to decrease costs, physicians and other providers compensated on a discounted fee-for-service basis may not cooperate fully with such efforts. The effect of nurse triage on busy primary care physicians in this situation is to eliminate the "quick and easy" visits, leaving only the more intensive ones that take more time and effort. Thus, trying to do the "right" thing for patients ends up hurting the hospital and possibly the physicians. Doing the "right" thing for patients and physicians ends up hurting the hospital. Aligning economic incentives becomes important. That may mean developing different ways to pay providers in late stage 2 and early stage 3 markets, so that the entire system can do what is "right" for the patient and overall appropriate use of constrained resources. As the market matures to a stage 4 market, these demand management services are generally well developed, accepted, and considered necessary to financial success.

Conclusion

In conclusion, a few principles must be kept in mind. Demand is increasingly a dominant force in medical interventions. We have to live within budgetary limits; it is not possible to do all things for all people. Rational choices must be made, but this does not necessarily mean "rationing." Demand management and call centers with nurse telephone management do not deny or inappropriately limit access, but rather create more appropriate access. Patients need to be, and generally want to be, more involved in decision making as related to their care. The needs of all stakeholders must be considered, so that incentives can be aligned to make the whole process work for all. Successful implementation of such systems will require significant investment in information technology, but it is possible to do this incrementally over a few years in most cases. The particular interventions must be based on scientific, evidence-based guidelines and protocols developed both at an individual patient level and a population level. These must be developed, implemented, and maintained by physicians and other clinical providers because they are the ones with "expert" knowledge. All these efforts ensure that patients get all the information required to make the best decision early and get the most appropriate and effective care for their problem.

References

1. Greenlick MR, Freeborn DK, Gambill GL, et al. Determinants of medical care utilization: the role of the telephone in total medical care. *Med Care.* 1973;11:121–134.

2. Infante-Rivard C, Krieger M, Petitcler M, et al. A telephone support service to reduce medical care use among the elderly. *J Am Geriatr Soc.* 1988;36:306–311.

3. Lazarus IR. Medical call centers: an effective demand management strategy for providers and plans. *Manage Healthcare.* 1995;56:58–59.

4. The Self-Care Institute. *Demand Management: Definition, Concepts and Model.* Washington, DC: Partnership for Prevention; 1996.

5. Miller, KA, Miller, EK. *Making Sense of Managed Care, I: Building Blocks and Fundamentals.* Tampa, Fla: Hillsboro Printing; 1997.

6. Poole SR, Schmitt BD, Carruth T, et al. After-hours telephone coverage: the application of an area-wide telephone triage and advice system for pediatric practices. *Pediatrics.* 1993;92(5):670–679.

7. Connor JP. Nurse phone care: a new way of thinking. *Med Group Manage J.* March/April 1996:22–27.

8. Brown HP. Demand management emerging as the next evolution of utilization management. *Manage Care Perspectives.* August 1996:1–3.

9. Grandinetti D. Patient phone calls driving you crazy? *Med Econ.* June 1996:72–75.

10. Richards B. Telephone triage cuts costly ER visits. *Wall Street Journal.* October 24, 1995;B1:3.

11. Gamignani J. Demand management: dial-a-nurse. *Business Health.* 1996;14(7):50.

12. Coile RC. *The Five Stages of Managed Care: Strategies for Providers, HMOs, and Suppliers.* Chicago, Ill: Health Administration Press; 1997.

13. Gulanick M, Green M, Crutchfield C, et al. Telephone nursing in a general medicine ambulatory clinic. *Medsurg Nurs.* 1996;5(2):93–98,124.

Appendix

After developing a business plan and mission statement, existing resources must be evaluated to determine what needs to be replaced, upgraded, or added to support a call center. Some of these items are as follows.

Telephone System. Will the current phone system support the business plan? Is the current phone system compatible with integrated services delivery network (ISDN) and/or T-1 systems? Will it support automatic call distributor or remote agents? Will the system support intelligent routing? Telephone systems must be scalable because call centers are constantly changing as new programs are added or deleted and business plans are modified.

Data/Software Programs. Current software programs must be evaluated to determine if current programs will work in a call center environment? Will the hardware need to be updated for future use? Will current appointment scheduling software work in a networked environment? Can the software be customized to accommodate different customers and applications? Can nurse triage software be changed or medical information updated at the physician's office? When evaluating software, look for areas in which several applications use the same program. For example, directory lookup software may have a physician answering service module, call scheduling module, etc., in the same package. As with voice systems, data/software programs must be adaptable to a changing environment.

Interactive Voice Response. An IVR system will be needed in the call center as a front end for many of the applications. For example, if a customer is calling to get information about his or her insurance benefit plan, the IVR can help him or her get the right information without talking to an agent.

Voice Mail/Auto Attendant. This can be used as a front end for certain applications. Such a system gives customers better access to information and the option to leave a message. Messages should be reviewed often for follow-up.

Internet. This offers many possibilities for getting information out to the public. For instance, customers can communicate with the call center by clicking a button on their personal computer; and the agent can see what page the customer is on and direct the Internet user to other pages, if needed. Putting information on the Internet can save networking costs and agent time.

Computer Telephony Integration. Computer telephony integration (CTI) systems link voice, data, and messaging. CTI technology is vital in a large call volume situation to better economize call handling time. CTI can also involve complex integration of technologies in the call center and requires up-front planning and coordination of efforts to work successfully.

Remote Agents. Can voice/data equipment support remote agents? Does the phone company have ISDN service to agent's homes? Can server connection support "screen" pops? Can personnel work on their own without benefit of supervision? Who will support technology at the agent's home?

Fax. Customers must be able to send or receive written information, if needed. Agents need to be able to fax information from the personal computer.

Real Estate. Where is the best location for the call center? What businesses are competing for nursing staff or agent staff? The area must grow as programs are added to the call center and provide room for on-site training for agents and nurses. The call center must be in an area in which the local telephone company can support the technology within the central office.

Personnel. What is the unemployment rate in the area? Are there personnel within the organization who can make the transition to a call center? Personnel must be cross-trained in several areas of the call center to be better used. All agents will not have the same skill level and services must be staffed accordingly. Structure staff in-service is vital to the success of the call center.

Type of Facilities. Can the local central office support the technology, i.e., ISDN, T-1 redundant and alternate trunk routing? Can the central office provided caller line identification?

Reporting Packages. These must be able to get reports on call volumes, staffing, monitoring of lines and equipment. Information needs to be accessible online to monitor calls.

Reliability should always be a consideration when evaluating systems. When establishing your protocols, a disaster recovery plan must be established with personnel and vendor support. A call center must provide good, reliable customer support.

Standardization of vendor products should be a major factor when evaluating products. Because of the complexity of the call center, integration of different products and vendors should be kept to a minimum. Service issues and response times will be important factors and the fewer vendors to be called the better.

Management of the call center is as critical as the technology for its success. Some of the key issues in call center management are as follows.

Enhancing customer service
Cost containment
Using current technology
Using available resources, i.e., personnel, data, telephony
Efficient scheduling of workforce
Flexibility and customization of services
Call processes have to be carefully tested and planned on an ongoing basis.

Call centers are a marriage of technology, personnel, and service. They are also an efficient and economical way to improve customer service and to provide various services.

About the Authors

Boyd K. Honeycutt, MD, MBA, FACP, is Vice President, Medical Management, for NovantHealth in Winston-Salem, N.C.

Suellen Burke is the Telecom Manager for Novant Health Triad Region.

Integrating Heterogeneous Healthcare Call Centers

Karen M. Peschel, LPN; William C. Reed, FHIMSS, FCHIME; Krista Salter

It is common to encounter various call centers as one navigates one's way through a healthcare organization. Numerous call centers collectively provide access to services in healthcare organizations: an external customer is processed by a referral call center, an internal customer requests assistance from an information services (IS) help desk, and a customer attempts to determine an individual's extension number. Despite the unique aspects of these heterogeneous call centers, many share common elements such as convenient and rapid access, appropriate support staff, and comprehensive performance management. Such commonality presents opportunities for healthcare organizations to integrate their call centers.

This article will explore the aspects, issues, and strategies involved in integrating heterogeneous call centers within a large, geographically disperse healthcare organization. In addition, it will present such integration within the context of substantial acquisition activities. Specifically, the article will examine the evolution of the organization's call centers; its integration strategy, including site consolidation, performance management, and enabling technologies; and integration challenges, anticipated benefits, and planned direction.

Business Environment

Olsten Health Services (OHS) is a home health organization consisting of multiple lines of business (LOBs). Originating from a core of home health nursing, OHS has grown, through de novo strategies and prudent acquisitions, into a multibillion dollar, diverse organization. Today, OHS offers a balanced portfolio of services via its healthcare management model (Figure 3.1).

OHS has expanded to become the premier provider of home health services throughout North America, with approximately 500 branches throughout the United States and Canada. Its nursing and infusion services capabilities are provided by nearly 100,000 full-time and per diem healthcare professionals resulting in more than 6 million patient visits per year. Through its network

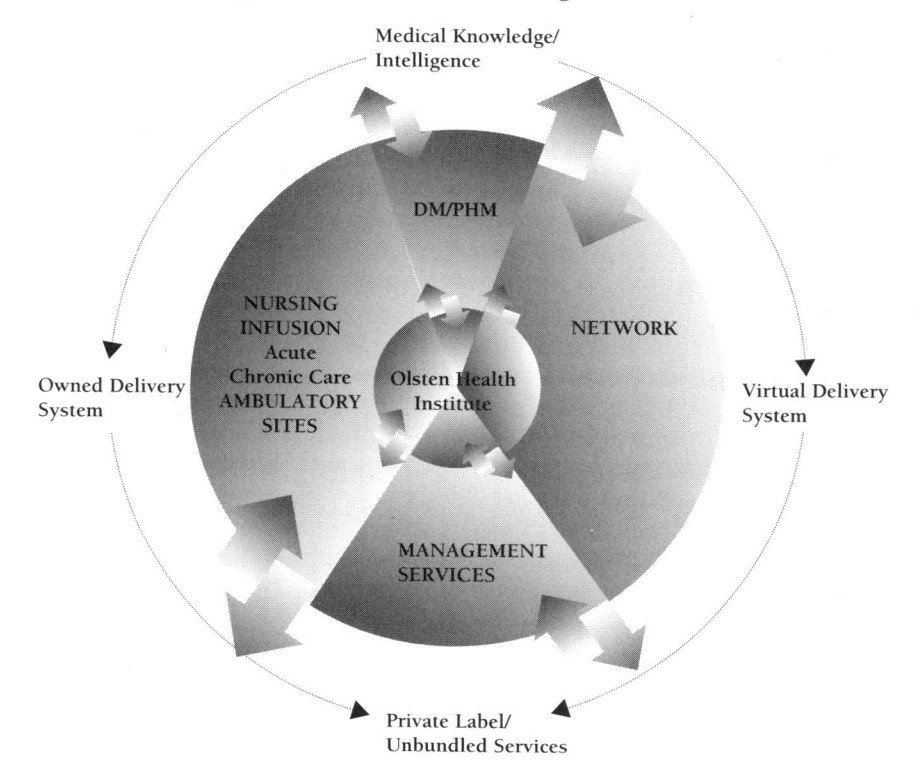

Figure 3.1. Healthcare Management Model

Medical Knowledge/Intelligence

DM/PHM

NURSING INFUSION
Acute
Chronic Care
AMBULATORY SITES

Olsten Health Institute

NETWORK

MANAGEMENT SERVICES

Owned Delivery System

Virtual Delivery System

Private Label/Unbundled Services

management LOB and a network of 3000 owned and subcontracted provider locations, OHS has alternate site healthcare management responsibility for over 20 million lives. With responsibility for such a range of healthcare services, OHS must depend on its call center capabilities to meet both customer and internal operating expectations.

Many of the segments of the OHS healthcare management model initially relied on one or more call centers. Because they were developed separately and at different times, most lacked a common management philosophy, consistent technology, or shared capabilities. In addition, as segments of this model grew, the associated acquisitions sometimes included similar and even competing call center capabilities. Thus, the growing dependency on call center capabilities, along with their heterogeneous nature, prompted OHS to evolve to a higher, more comprehensive, call center management philosophy.

Call Center Evolution

In 1997, OHS operated five different types of call centers in 18 separate locations. The genesis and characteristics of those call centers are as follows.

National Resource Center. The National Resource Center (NRC) was the OHS's first foray into the call center environment. This department, part of a 1992 home care acquisition, was originally envisioned as a customer support department focusing on national account customers. National account referral sources access the toll-free number to make service requests, query service capabilities, and discuss account pricing. Available Monday through Friday 8 AM to 8 PM Eastern Time, the NRC is staffed by both clinical and nonclinical coordinators. The NRC also works with the Departments of Sales, Strategic Planning, and Marketing Communications by responding to calls generated from multimedia initiatives. These calls include employment inquiries, brochure requests, and general program/service inquiries.

Today, although this department retains its original vision, its mission has expanded to include customer complaint management and specialty program support. In addition, the NRC has become an important resource for internal customers, providing information about contracts and pricing, programs and services, and general resources. In 1997, the NRC responded to more than 40,000 inbound calls from internal and external customers.

Clinical Support Desk. As part of an infusion services company acquisition, OHS became responsible for the clinical support desk (CSD). The CSD is a 24-hour, seven-day-per-week telephonic clinical support capability staffed by nurses. The CSD was formed to provide three fundamental services. First, it was intended to serve as a clinical reference center to assist patients and physicians with questions and issues related to specific and unique therapies used in treating problems such as primary pulmonary hypertension, amyotrophic lateral sclerosis, etc. Second, the CSD served as an intake site for patients requiring access to some of these therapies. Finally, since the CSD was required to be available 24 hours a day, seven days per week for other reasons, it was determined to use the CSD for off-hours clinical calls for infusion services issues. Historically, these calls were handled by multiple answering services which then paged on-call clinicians. In 1997, 140,000 calls were placed to the CSD.

Central Intake Centers. Several large "central" intake centers were also part of a home care acquisition. These sites are responsible for intake and insurance verification for all referrals within a defined geographic area. Standard hours of operation are 8 AM to 6 PM Monday through Friday, but some sites have expanded hours due to high referral volume. All sites are staffed by nurses and reimbursement specialists. Currently, OHS has 10 such central intake centers. The technology at these central intake centers is varied based on history and size, with four using Nortel private branch exchange (PBX) technology and automated call distribution (ACD) technology and the remaining sites using key systems with no ACD support.

Regional Network Centers. In 1996, OHS opened the first of five regional network centers (RNCs). These sites were created to provide managed care customers a single source for centralized intake and billing, quality assurance, and data reporting and analysis. These sites also offer home care case management by coordinating services with local providers either directly through OHS branch operations or through a network of high-quality subcontractors, thus managing utilization. In 1997, OHS RNCs responded to more than 340,000 inbound calls.

Help Desk. Internally, the OHS IS provides a geographically diverse communications network supporting the 500 sites running multiple applications in various technical environments distributed and centralized in Overland Park, Kansas. The internal customer support mechanism that assists with technical problems is the IS Help Desk, also located in Overland Park. This call center is staffed 10 hours per day, five days per week, with off-hours calls being answered by an automated attendant with associated automated paging for critical incidents. Because of the varied technical platforms within each LOB, five queues have been established in the ACD environment, each geared to supporting a specific LOB. Reporting is generated within the Telecorp management tool to provide the call center manager with the ability to monitor the performance of each LOB support queue. During 1997, the Help Desk responded to more than 130,000 calls.

Integration Strategy

All of these various OHS call centers evolved independently, with virtually no common coordination or oversight. While they frequently represented duplicative operations and resources, there was little commonality in standards, processes, or technologies. At times, they even presented competing services which only confused and frustrated customers. It became apparent that enhanced customer satisfaction and reduced operating expense would only be possible through a fundamental shift in the management philosophy regarding OHS call centers. Thus, having assessed the situation, OHS senior management recognized the need to have a different call center operating model and embarked on a method to define an integrated version. Figure 3.2 depicts the methodology being used, along with the associated integration strategy with its five strategic initiatives.

To facilitate the transition to a new model, the first strategic initiative was the creation of a new position, i.e., Director of Access Services. This position, whether through direct management responsibility or indirect coordination, ensures satisfactory customer (internal and external) access to all OHS services. The Director of Access Services defines standard operating philosophies and processes; helps OHS call center performance management expectations evolve, which includes customer service targets, operational performance metrics, and associated measurement and reporting; and identifies enabling technologies to be used.

Once the Director of Access Services position was defined, a set of three other initiatives began simultaneously to structure the framework for an integrated call center model. The second initiative is the assessment of site con-

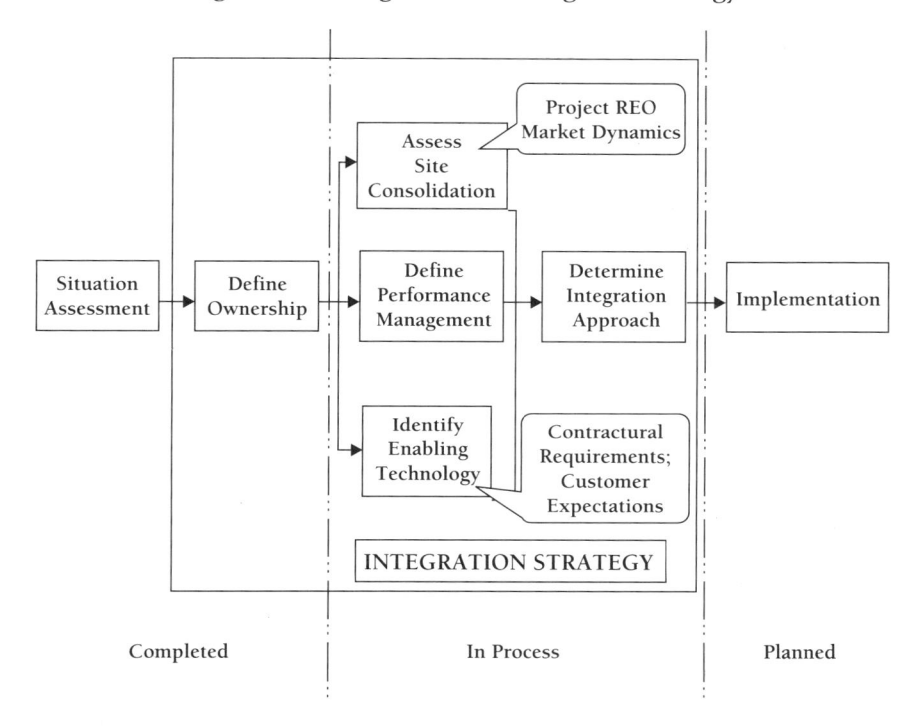

Figure 3.2. Integration Planning Methodology

```
Situation     →  Define       →  [Assess Site Consolidation]  ← Project REO Market Dynamics
Assessment       Ownership       Define Performance Management → Determine Integration Approach → Implementation
                                 Identify Enabling Technology ← Contractual Requirements; Customer Expectations

                                 INTEGRATION STRATEGY

Completed        |           In Process                |        Planned
```

solidation options. The following market dynamics are being considered during this assessment:

- Market demographics for the sites being assessed
- Domain expertise to be replaced in the event of employee turnover
- Labor pool characteristics and availability at the consolidated site(s)
- Potential performance improvement/economies of scale

In addition, OHS has simultaneously initiated a significant effort to reengineer enterprise operations (dubbed "Project REO"). One component of Project REO, led by the Director of Access Services, is to establish an enterprise-wide approach to customer access rather than the silo approach historically used by LOB. Obviously, the results and recommendations from this Project REO effort will help to craft any final consolidation decisions.

The third strategic initiative involves the definition and dissemination of operating performance expectations, providing a framework within which call centers can operate. This initiative is coupled with the provision of consistent measurement and management reporting.

The fourth strategic initiative is the identification, acquisition, and implementation of consistent call center enabling technology. From call receipt (which perhaps includes caller identification) to database interaction to call resolution, this technology will assist in processing and managing all calls received by the integrated call centers. Where appropriate and feasible, the technology will also be integrated to encompass both telephony and information management.

Once complete, the outcomes from these three initiatives will converge to provide input to the final strategic initiative, determining the appropriate integration approach which will result in call center services that enhance overall customer capabilities while reducing unnecessary operational overhead.

Site Consolidation. Site consolidation involves consideration of three specific dimensions. First, the appropriate combination of existing centralized call centers into more regional/national integrated call centers will be evaluated based on the various market dynamics previously noted. Related to these decisions is the second dimension, i.e., how RNCs and centralized call centers could be consolidated when an enterprise-wide focus is taken instead of an LOB perspective.

The third dimension involves the unique capabilities provided by national call centers such as the NRC and CSD. Commonality of functions, staff, and technologies indicates that the consolidation of these functions would be prudent. These two sites currently have a national focus and extended hours of operation. In addition, they are highly dependent on technology to support their operations and are in dire need of upgraded system support. Each site also has immediate space constraints with limited room to expand.

Performance Management. The establishment of the RNCs and their associated contractual commitments to defined call responses was a key driver in the decision to invest in ACD and reporting technology. While the use of ACD monitoring was routine in some parts of the healthcare industry, this type of performance management was new to home care. In 1995, OHS received its first contract which mandated adherence to telephone service standards. At that time, the only OHS call center to monitor call volume was the NRC, with no automation to facilitate the process. The manager was required to manually aggregate raw data from the telephone switch to determine call volume. There were no defined standards against which to measure and monitor performance.

In 1996, in response to customer mandates, senior management sponsored an initiative to identify and implement an ACD reporting package at all RNCs. Telecorp was eventually selected as the ACD vendor for OHS. Call center metrics were established based on industry standards and on feedback received from OHS customers. OHS performance goals were established for 90 percent of calls to be answered within 30 seconds, with a lost call rate not to exceed 5 percent. A standard set of reports was identified and the ACD at each RNC was configured to generate these reports daily. Each RNC site manager is responsible for reviewing and communicating the data to the staff. On a monthly basis, each site sends data to Access Services where it is aggregated and formatted for senior management review.

The Telecorp product also contains a module, Agent Window, which allows real-time monitoring of ACD queues. The personal computer–based system feeds reader boards throughout the call center, which allows a call center manager to monitor real-time queue activity through both the personal computer and reader board. Thus, while not truly "proactive," the reader boards at least offer an early warning system to facilitate queue balancing.

Performance metrics and ACD reporting are now in place at all OHS call centers except the central intake centers. Access Services is responsible for the coordination, training, analysis, and support required to ensure that each location has appropriate queue allocation and all of the resources needed to successfully meet the OHS performance management goals.

Enabling Technology. A significant challenge for the OHS call centers is the lack of standardized, technically sophisticated systems. Each of the call centers originally employed multiple, nonintegrated information technology. To become successfully integrated, clearly this needed to change. So OHS embarked on a multipronged approach to integrate its call center information technologies.

Following an internally developed, structured method referred to as the Healthcare Information Architecture, OHS first standardized its telephony, employing both switching technology and voice mail from Nortel. This standardization not only enabled seamless call center communications, but also supported transparent call transfers among the call centers, field branches, and corporate support locations. The Nortel products are the foundation on which the framework of call center management has been built

Next, OHS began to examine the applications portfolio that supported its various call centers. In 1993, the NRC had replaced manual call processing with an internally developed Windows-based program written in a programming language known as Clipper. In 1994, the system was enhanced to support "live" online call processing using patient zip codes to locate appropriate service providers. Once processed, the referral service request is then sent to the provider branch, via fax server, for handling. The need for fast, accurate data entry was becoming a priority as call volume increased and the department expanded to meet the needs of OHS customers. The Clipper system was proving to be inflexible and inadequate to support the information requirements of this expanding department.

Conversely, the CSD had multiple applications supporting its processes. The Centramax system from National Health Enhancement Systems was implemented to support the CSD's triage function, which included call follow-up. For access to patient records, the CSD used two internally developed systems, Patient Record Information System Management (PRISM), used to support the infusion LOB, and Medical Electronic Data System (MEDS), for access to nursing service patients. Unfortunately, these applications were not integrated, which necessitated call center operators to be conversant with multiple technical platforms.

The central intake centers are, for the most part, manual; however, four sites use front-end data entry screens developed for MEDS. The systems are laborious and cumbersome at best, were not integrated, and lacked comprehensive connectivity with the CSD.

The RNCs are supported by yet another information system, NETWOR$_X$, which was converted from a commercially available system. NETWOR$_X$ has some distinct advantages over the other call center systems in that it uses more current technology and integrates all five RNCs through a common database.

Finally, the IS Help Desk, because of its unique, nonclinical nature, uses a stand-alone system known as case-based reasoning (CBR). This system is accessible across the OHS wide area network so that the remote regional technicians throughout the country can query and update statuses of various system problems.

As OHS sought to integrate its call centers, this collection of disparate systems obviously presented an enormous challenge. To addresses this challenge, two initiatives were pursued. First, as an interim measure, IS used its data transformation management system to foster intrasystem communications. Such integration provides single point-of-data capture, facilitated communication via e-mail and desktop faxing, and broader information access and visibility throughout the call centers. However, true call center integration can only be achieved through fundamental process change. Thus, the reengineering process within Project REO will establish an enterprise-wide approach to call center information management rather than the disparate systems historically employed. It is anticipated that this reengineering will lead to the implementation of a single (except for the IS Help Desk) integrated call center IS.

Integration Challenges

Perhaps the most challenging integration issue is goal alignment. Due to the assorted expectations represented by varied LOBs, which is exacerbated by different philosophies encountered during acquisitions, common goal alignment is extremely difficult. The fundamental goals are not very different, but the expectations for the goals and the path to achieve them are radically different.

A second integration challenge exists with regard to site consolidation. While site consolidation represents clear opportunities for reducing operating expenses and expanding coverage and services, corporate knowledge is in dire jeopardy. Lacking any degree of sophistication in enabling technology, much of the call centers' corporate knowledge is contained in the minds of the individuals that staff them. That knowledge has evolved through training and experience over a period of years. Retention and replacement of that knowledge during site consolidation are the paramount concerns of integration planning.

Technology conversion offers significant challenges as well. Being somewhat antiquated because of their origins in prior acquired organizations, many of the call centers' supporting technologies lack the flexibility to easily migrate to more state-of-the-art standardized platforms. In addition, their lack of sophistication (and in many instances, documentation) requires an extremely close relationship with their users to create the corporate knowledge and capabilities previously discussed. This cybernetic relationship will be extremely fragile as both technologies and staff are replaced.

User management offers other challenges. Rapid company growth, whether through business growth or acquisitions, accompanied by high turnover, creates an environment in which it is difficult to keep call center operators adequately trained. Although it is desirable to have users focus only on the functional aspects of information technology, increasing complexity of call center technology is requiring operators (or at least someone in the call center) to have a rudimentary understanding of the technical aspects of the systems. Furthermore, balancing call center resources to meet performance expectations is a complex task involving business acumen, knowledge of queuing theory, and some luck. Appropriate understanding and utilization of the OHS ACD systems and their associated queues is a daunting task which requires significant further refinement.

In addition, the national scope of OHS call centers requires close attention and adherence to a broad set of clinical policy practice issues in telemedicine/telehealth. Unfortunately, the absence of firm national guidelines regarding practice standards for clinical call centers makes it a challenge to provide such attention. The National Council of State Boards of Nursing[1] is currently exploring the idea of multistate licensure, which, by endorsement, would give nurses the legal authority to practice in participating states without obtaining individual state licenses. Known as "mutual recognition,"[2] it would enable nurses to hold a license in one state and practice in any participating state, provided that they adhere to the specific laws and regulations of the state in which they are providing clinical service. Under the auspices of the Department of Health and Human Services, the Joint Working Group on Telemedicine, a group charged with developing national policies on telemedicine and reporting the findings to Vice President Al Gore and Congress, is also searching for ways to reduce cross-state licensure barriers for providers.[1] In 1997, the American Association of Ambulatory Care Nursing (AAACN) acknowledged the "vital role that telephone nursing practice plays in delivering professional nursing care to patients in a variety of settings" by releasing the first guidelines on telephone nursing practice.[3] The AAACN views the document as "the 'starting point' of an evolutionary process for these standards of practice."[3] OHS continually monitors such initiatives in its pursuit of the highest standards of clinical practice.

Finally, a common fundamental challenge exists with regard to transition, i.e., how to migrate to the new model while maintaining adequate service to existing customers. Due to the critical nature of healthcare services, this challenge is even more acute than in most service organizations.

Anticipated Benefits

OHS goals of customer service, quality, employee satisfaction, and reasonable cost help achieve expected benefits of call center integration. Even from a virtual perspective, integration has already produced improved customer and employee satisfaction. Customers are encountering single points of contact and realizing consistent levels of performance. Internally, employees now function in an environment of defined performance expectations and supportive enabling technologies, where their participation in corporate knowledge represents a contribution rather than a dependency.

This new integrated environment will enable OHS to develop its healthcare management model with optimal transparency to its customers. Consistent philosophies, processes, and technologies will allow customers to navigate among the various model segments in a seamless manner. The new call center environment will also position OHS to evolve to a future state of expanded direct patient communication and interaction via integrated voice, data, and video communications.

Planned Direction

Today, OHS finds itself in a position to use all the experience gained in its existing call centers and use it to build its model for the future. Several significant initiatives are under way to enable the future to be realized.

First, the reengineering of OHS call center operations to incorporate an enterprise-wide view will produce an operating model for the future which maximizes customer satisfaction while minimizing associated operating costs. This complex team initiative will be completed in phases through 1999.

Next, planning is under way to consolidate two existing sites, the NRC and the CSD, into one expanded national call center. The proposed consolidated call center will offer a portfolio of three specific services. First, it will provide intake and referral processing services similar to those provided by the NRC today. Second, the clinical (telemedicine) support provided by the CSD will be perpetuated in this new, consolidated model. Third, recognizing the logical progression to more direct interaction and communication with homebound patients, this new call center will also have the capability to provide clinical telemonitoring (telehealth) and data recording 24 hours a day, seven days per week. This consolidated call center will be housed in the new OHS corporate services center in Overland Park, Kansas, which is currently under construction. Proximity to IS should ensure immediate on-site systems and telecommunications support.

Finally, as OHS evolves its enterprise-wide customer access model, commensurate integrated information capabilities will be identified, developed, and implemented to support it. Disparate labor-intensive systems will be replaced by functionally robust, integrated capabilities that facilitate customer interaction, use single point-of-data capture, ensure balanced operations, and provide insightful management reporting.

Only through the successful convergence of these three initiatives can such system integration occur and the OHS call centers achieve their optimal levels of performance. The ultimate goal is to create a customer-focused call center environment that will support the mission and vision of OHS.

Summary

In a relatively short period, OHS has absorbed multiple call centers supporting different LOBs from various acquisitions, functioning with diverse standards, processes, and technologies. However, customer and employee satisfaction is predicated on OHS's ability to thoroughly integrate these heterogeneous call centers.

The integration was initiated and has successfully progressed through a balanced program of focused leadership and a defined strategy which includes site consolidation, sound performance management philosophies, and enabling technology. Benefits have already been achieved with even more substantive ones to occur as the integration continues to evolve.

References

1. Granade PF. The brave new world of telemedicine. *RN.* 1997;60(7):59–62.
2. Susman ES. Nursing boards to work for reciprocal licensing. *Telemed Virtual Reality.* 1997;2(12):2–12.
3. American Academy of Ambulatory Care Nursing. *Telephone Nursing Practice Administration and Practice Standards: 1997.* Pitman, NJ: Anthony J. Jannetti Inc; 1997.

Suggested Readings

Appleby C. Speed dialing. *Hosp Health Networks.* 1997;71(10):59–60.
Chin T. Call centers improve service, carry out managed care goals. *Health Data Manage.* 1998;6(2):122–131.
Hammer M, Champy J. *Reengineering the Corporation: A Manifesto for Business Revolution.* New York, NY: Harper Business; 1994.
Hiatt J. *Winning with Quality.* Reading, Mass: Addison-Wesley Longman; 1995.
Lawson C. Is your help desk ready for disaster? *Teleprofessional.* 1997;10(5):68–70,90–96.
Ousey A. Call center technology to the rescue. *Call Center Magazine.* 1997;10(11):89–96.
Medical Education and Council on Medical Service. *The Promotion of Quality Telemedicine.* (Resolution 309, I–95, Resolves 1–3); CME/CMS Report A–96. 1996.
Mikol T. Progress towards a customer interaction center. *Telemarketing Call Center Solutions.* 1997;16(4):70–81.

About the Authors

Karen M. Peschel, LPN, is Director of Access and Data Integrity Services for Olsten Health Services in Natick, Massachusetts.

William C. Reed, FHIMSS, FCHIME, is Senior Vice President, Information and Administrative Services for Olsten Health Services in Melville, New York.

Krista Salter is Manager of Voice Services for Olsten Health Services in Overland Park, Kansas.

Managing Care Through High-Quality, Customer-Focused Service: HealthCall

Mary Ann Baxter; Pamela S. Blankenship; Edward Kornacki; Cathy McMahan; Bill Epstein

Background

Blue Cross Blue Shield of Michigan (BCBSM) is the largest Blue Cross plan in the country and the dominant healthcare provider in Michigan. BCBSM and its affiliate company, the Blue Care Network (BCN), provide a full spectrum of health services and products ranging from traditional health insurance to exciting new blended managed care/traditional products. Michigan has a total population of 9.3 million people of which 4.4 million are BCBSM members. Within Michigan, 75 percent of the population has been, is, or will be a BCBSM member.

The mission of BCBSM is to excel in the delivery of healthcare-related products and services that emphasize access to quality healthcare at affordable prices. BCBSM is committed to meeting its public responsibilities and maintaining its nonprofit status.

However, in spite of its tremendous success, the company faces many competitive challenges as it moves forward. As indicated by Richard Whitmer, President and Chief Executive Officer of BCBSM, in the 1996 Annual Report, Blue Cross must change to survive: "As a major force in an industry going through wrenching change, BCBSM is transforming the way it does business to meet the demands of a market in upheaval.... Our competitive challenge is that other insurers, some from out of state and many of them well-financed, are planning to enter the Michigan market and convert our traditional membership to their managed care plans. Our response is to strengthen our managed care products ... through integrated health management (IHM)."

The goal of IHM is to manage the total health experience of healthcare consumers throughout the continuum of care. IHM has redefined healthcare to include health education, prevention, and professional care management, tying all of these elements together in an integrated approach to health and health maintenance (Figure 4.1).

In 1995, BCBSM began developing the base components of the IHM programs. The demand management system, HealthCall, a telephone-based healthcare service, was implemented on July 1, 1997. This service provides 24–hour-a-day, seven–day-a-week access to a licensed registered nurse and medical information.

This case study will address the evolution of the BCBSM HealthCall Center and answer the following questions.

- Why was this solution chosen?
- How was this service implemented?
- What has been its impact thus far, and do demand management systems affect healthcare consumption?

To answer these questions we will review the design of the service, the software development effort, the identification of resources and staffing, and the implementation of this product.

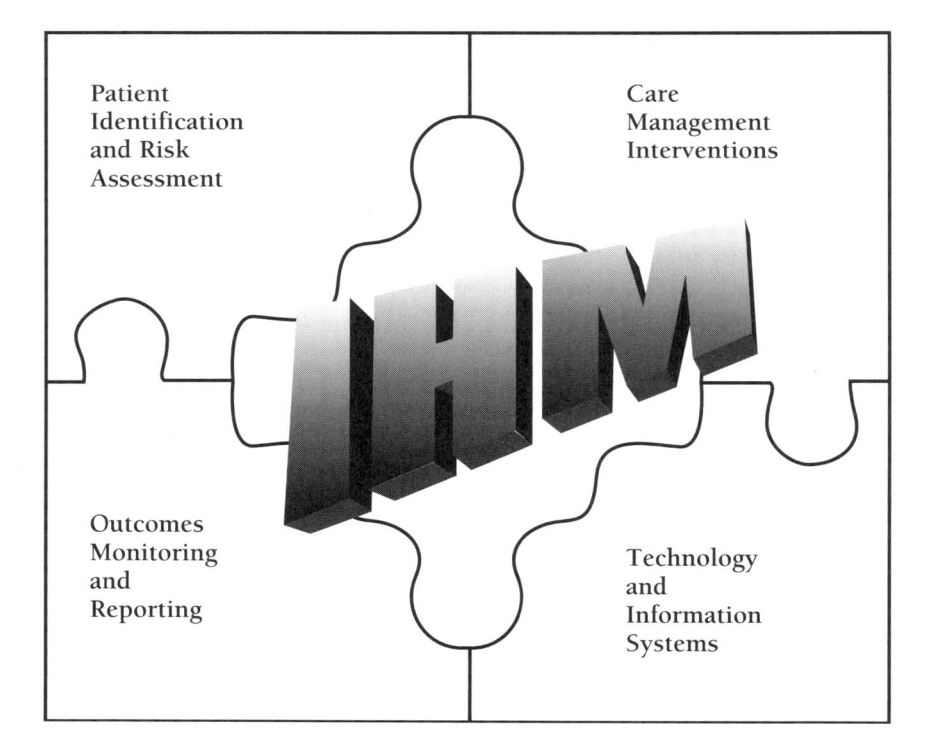

Figure 4.1. Integrated Health Management Vision

Source: BlueCross BlueShield of Michigan. Used by permission.

The Marketplace

Healthcare has traditionally been an industry in which provider interventions focused on acute care for the patient when the patient entered the healthcare system because of a health-related episode. The insurer's perspective focused on financial considerations, primarily claims payment and billing. In this fee-for-service world, physicians, facilities, and specialists operated relatively freely to provide the care that was deemed necessary and agreed to by the patient. Insurers acted after the fact to pay for services. Competition was based primarily on price and a standard variety of coverage offerings. Most activities in this environment were reactive and retrospective.

In today's environment, the focus is shifting from reactive and retrospective to proactive and prospective. The key health industry changes are as follows.

- Healthcare delivery is changing from episode-based care to one of prevention, wellness, and the provision of services across the full continuum of care potentially over the lifetime of the member.
- Healthcare orientation is shifting from a concentration on the treatment provided to a focus on the outcomes achieved by the treatments used.
- Consumers are now participating in preserving health and treatment planning through a shared decision-making process.
- Healthcare's central focus is shifting from treatment of an illness to preservation of wellness.
- Utilization management is changing from retrospective to concurrent and prospective review.

The Problem

Historically, BCBSM had concentrated on managing healthcare wherever a patient had an encounter with the healthcare system. The management role in this process was to impose administrative controls on the provider in an attempt to control utilization and cost. While this approach did address cost issues, it did not support the consumer and coordinate the entire healthcare experience to improve the delivery of service and the quality of care. Consequently, consumers were left on their own to identify the services they required and manage the delivery of healthcare from various providers. Unfortunately, consumers rarely have the healthcare information and experience required for effectively managing and coordinating care. For chronic or long-term illness, consumers must ensure that all their healthcare providers are working together and coordinating the management of the disease and the delivery of service. In emergencies, they are forced to make medical assessments and determine the appropriate solution with little or no real healthcare expertise.

The result, of course, is that the consumer receives poorly managed healthcare. Duplicate services are provided, contradictory management plans are employed, and healthcare services are inappropriately used. Consumers, operating with little or no healthcare expertise, are often left to fend for themselves in this confusing and complex environment.

BCBSM Response

To provide healthcare consumers with the knowledge they require and the support they need to manage their total healthcare experience, BCBSM developed the IHM strategy. The focus of the IHM managed care products is to:

- Achieve better healthcare outcomes.
- Increase the satisfaction of consumers and providers.
- Reduce medical risks and costs.
- Lower administrative costs and increase revenue.

IHM redefines healthcare to include health education, prevention, and professional care management, tying all these elements together in an integrated approach to healing and health maintenance. It is based on three simple but powerful ideas.

Health is not a thing we have or do not have, but an ongoing state or continuum ranging from complete wellness to terminal illness.
With appropriate education, people can take steps to keep themselves in the wellness part of the continuum, preserving health and fitness through lifestyle improvements.
When illness strikes, care can be managed cost-effectively to achieve the best results for the member and provide high-quality care.

IHM is a fully integrated process for managing the total health experience of the healthcare consumer throughout the continuum of care. This strategy consists of demand management, disease management, and utilization management.

Demand Management. The first component of the IHM strategy is the front-end of the health/illness continuum with services related to maintaining health and wellness. This component is primarily a consumer-based health management approach focusing on preventing illness, assessing member risk, and helping members make informed decisions on the level of treatment required.

Disease Management. The second component of the IHM strategy is disease or medical management. This is a comprehensive approach to managing the care needs of a patient with selected diseases or conditions across the entire healthcare delivery system and throughout the life cycle of a disease.

Utilization Management. The third component of the IHM strategy is utilization management, which refers to initiatives focused on the provider and the manner in which healthcare services are supplied. Utilization management strives to ensure that services are medically appropriate and provided efficiently.

IHM Demand Management. The foundation of the IHM initiative is HealthCall, a demand management program that provides members with telephone access to licensed registered nurses and medical information 24 hours a day, seven days a week. The primary goal of HealthCall is to offer the consumer direct access to expert clinical information. The expected outcome of providing this information is that customers will make better choices in the healthcare services that they use.

When individuals lack access to health information, they frequently choose higher-cost treatment. Studies conducted by leading research organizations estimate that at least 32 percent of emergency room visits do not require urgent medical care and about 40 percent of all health services may, to some extent, be unnecessary.

The Design and Development of the HealthCall Program

Program Design. BCBSM's HealthCall program provides a single infrastructure for the coordination and delivery of medical and member services (Figure 4.2). The first requirement in building the HealthCall program was to determine the services that would be provided and the best delivery for each service. The primary goal was to provide clinical information to the consumer. The key components required to achieve this goal are as follows.

Medical Condition Triage. The HealthCall service had to respond to customers seeking advice for medical symptoms. The inquiries could range from relatively insignificant complaints to life-threatening conditions. The service had to deliver high-quality, consistent recommendations that were clinically and legally sound. Therefore, two essential components of the HealthCall service were designed to ensure that these requirements were met.

1. The HealthCall nurse: HealthCall nurses are required to have a broad range of clinical experience. Their clinical background must ensure that they can handle any type of medical symptoms with which they are confronted. The nurses are trained in telephone triage and are required to undergo simulated HealthCall exercises as the final stage of their training. Within HealthCall, the nurse is the ultimate clinical authority who ensures that the clinical recommendations are appropriate for the patient's medical history and current symptoms.
2. The medical algorithms: The HealthCall medical algorithms ensure the delivery of consistent medical recommendations. The algorithms provide the nurse with recommendations on the level of care required, the precautions that should be taken, and the follow-up care required. The recommendations are based on patient demographics and reported symptoms.

Healthcare Information. The HealthCall service offers the consumer the following ways to gather information related to particular medical questions.

Figure 4.2. Blue Cross Blue Shield of Michigan HealthCall Infrastructure

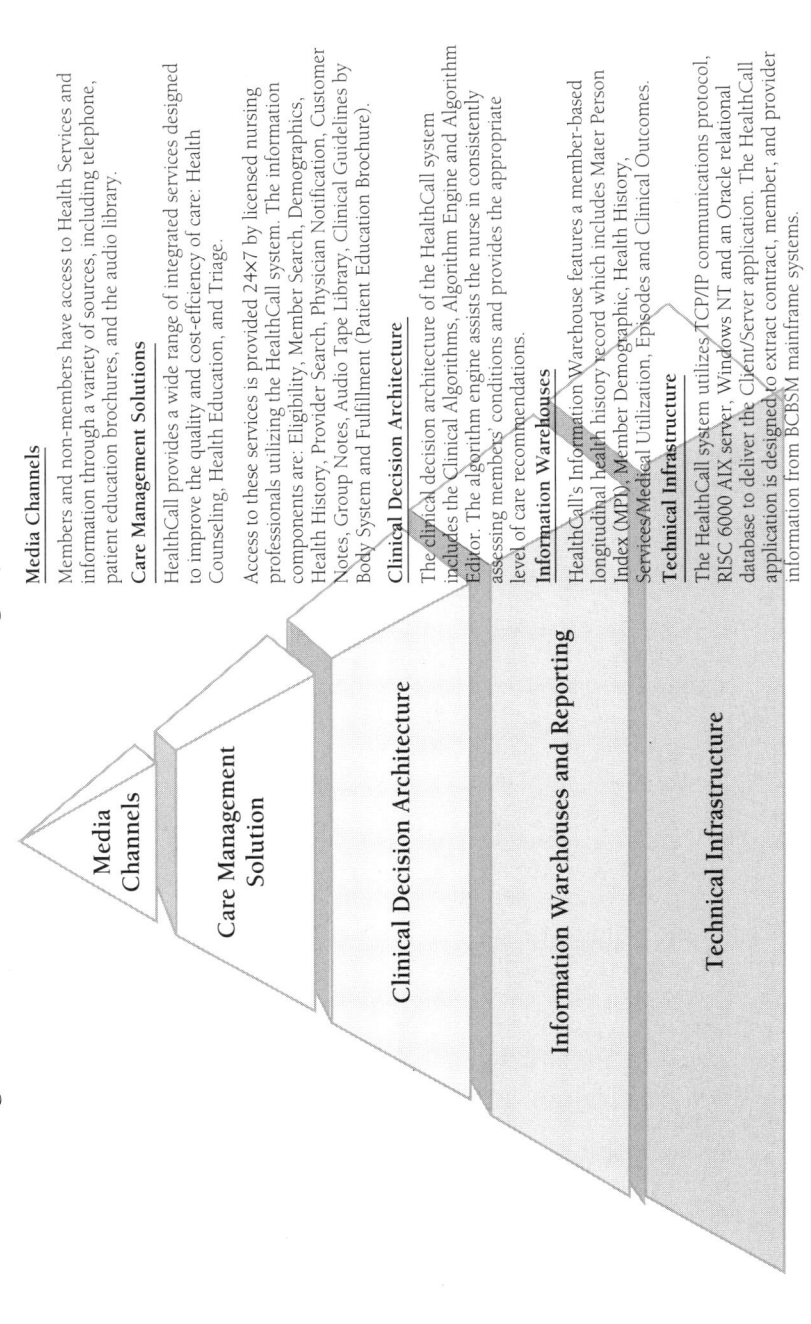

Media Channels

Members and non-members have access to Health Services and information through a variety of sources, including telephone, patient education brochures, and the audio library.

Care Management Solutions

HealthCall provides a wide range of integrated services designed to improve the quality and cost-efficiency of care: Health Counseling, Health Education, and Triage.

Access to these services is provided 24x7 by licensed nursing professionals utilizing the HealthCall system. The information components are: Eligibility, Member Search, Demographics, Health History, Provider Search, Physician Notification, Customer Notes, Group Notes, Audio Tape Library, Clinical Guidelines by Body System and Fulfillment (Patient Education Brochure).

Clinical Decision Architecture

The clinical decision architecture of the HealthCall system includes the Clinical Algorithms, Algorithm Engine and Algorithm Editor. The algorithm engine assists the nurse in consistently assessing members' conditions and provides the appropriate level of care recommendations.

Information Warehouses

HealthCall's Information Warehouse features a member-based longitudinal health history record which includes Mater Person Index (MPI), Member Demographic, Health History, Services/Medical Utilization, Episodes and Clinical Outcomes.

Technical Infrastructure

The HealthCall system utilizes TCP/IP communications protocol, RISC 6000 AIX server, Windows NT and an Oracle relational database to deliver the Client/Server application. The HealthCall application is designed to extract contract, member, and provider information from BCBSM mainframe systems.

Source: BlueCross BlueShield of Michigan. Used by permission.

1. Health education guidelines: These offer a broad range of clinical information on numerous common health questions. The guidelines cover the medical signs and symptoms, common preventive measures that can be taken, treatment options, and potential medical outcomes.
2. Informational Brochures: The customer can receive a number of brochures discussing common medical conditions. These brochures describe the condition, precautions, and preventive health guidelines; recommendations on medical screening; and answers to the most frequently asked questions.
3. Audio health library: This library contains prerecorded tapes on different medical topics ranging from specific conditions related to a given age group to general health questions. The customer may chose to go directly to the audio health library and select the topics desired or the nurse may use this service to respond to an educational question.
4. Preventive service reminders: The HealthCall system contains various preventive health reminders. During the course of a telephone call, the system will alert a nurse to review a preventive health issue with the customer. The system will send the nurse reminder messages when the specified demographic criteria are met. For instance, if a mother is calling about a young child, the system may remind the nurse to review the required infant immunizations.
5. Customized medical information searches: The HealthCall program offers the nurse several options in providing clinical information on unusual topics or inquiries. The online system includes a 27–volume medical reference library which allows the nurse to rapidly look up any medication, symptom, or disease. The medical librarian may use the Internet or the medical library to develop a detailed research paper on any healthcare topic requested.

Provider Directory, Referral, and Notification. The HealthCall service offers the following types of information on providers and their locations.
1. Physician referral: The HealthCall nurse may assist the customer in locating a provider by searching the BCBSM provider network using various search criteria.
2. Facilities: The HealthCall nurse may direct a customer to the facility that offers the specific service required, one that their physician is affiliated with, or search for facilities based on various search criteria.
3. Community resources: The HealthCall nurse may provide information to the customer related to community resources based on the location of the customer and the type of resource or support organization requested.
4. Primary care physician (PCP) communication: The HealthCall system automatically notifies a member's PCP, via an automated fax letter, whenever a member is directed to seek urgent or emergency care.

Workflow Management. The HealthCall system employs a workflow component which allows HealthCall users to manage and route work across the department. The individual user may schedule and route work activities as needed, and the HealthCall management may administer work for specific individuals or groups of users.

In addition to these services, BCBSM wanted the capability to evaluate and measure both the operational efficiency and the impact on the customer of the HealthCall service. The measurements would need to provide feedback on customer satisfaction, the quality of the clinical evaluation and recommendations, and the impact on the utilization of healthcare services. Therefore, the system had to be capable of conducting customer satisfaction surveys and correlate with member claims data. Additional performance feedback would also be provided by customer satisfaction surveys performed by independent researchers.

Buy Versus Build. Several alternatives were considered in the development of the HealthCall service. In today's market, a vendor may be hired to supply the service requested, a packaged solution may be purchased, or a custom application developed. BCBSM chose to develop a custom application for the following reasons.

- Integration with existing BCBSM systems would ensure that membership and provider updates were coordinated with the main BCBSM systems at all times.
- Clinical information and recommendations would be designed to conform to existing BCBSM and BCN guidelines and requirements, thus providing consistency in the clinical information supplied throughout BCBSM and BCN.
- Customer-specific requests and requirements could be easily supported by integrating with existing services to implement and maintain such requests.
- The impact on healthcare utilization could be evaluated by the linkage between HealthCall usage and BCBSM and BCN utilization experience.

Meeting the Challenges

Numerous challenges had to be overcome to successfully implement HealthCall and IHM as a whole, the most important ones being technology, "24 x 7" support, and implementation.

Technology. The IHM strategy required BCBSM to move to a new technological plateau. The existing BCBSM technical environment consisted primarily of legacy mainframe systems. Given this infrastructure, several obstacles stood in the path of the successful implementation of the HealthCall service. The technology used for the HealthCall application was still relatively new to BCBSM. Although there were minor client/server applications in production, only one other major client/server application was implemented before HealthCall. The technical support organization was built to maintain the existing mainframe technologies. The infrastructure required to support new client/server technologies was just emerging within BCBSM.

To overcome this obstacle BCBSM worked closely with IBM to secure technical expertise in client/server design and development, as well as expertise in business process design for nurse call centers. This partnership resulted in the development of the HealthCall customer relationship management model (Figure 4.3), which provides a technical architecture to support HealthCall both now and in the future. To develop this architecture IBM used the rapid application development technique. This approach allowed both the technical team to move forward quickly and the user team to begin developing training strategies, policies, and procedures, and hiring staff. The subsequent HealthCall system is a two-tier client/server application developed in Visual Basic 5.0, with an Oracle database running on a UNIX AIX server and using a Windows NT 4.0 client.

24 x 7 Support. The delivery of services required expansion of the system's availability. BCBSM has a number of applications, which run 24 hours a day, seven days a week. However, HealthCall was the first 24 x 7 application that had users on-site around the clock. Consequently, support mechanisms had to be developed to ensure that the users could get support for problems with networks, applications, telephones, or building facilities whenever it was needed.

To overcome this obstacle BCBSM appointed an Information Systems Technical Coordinator for the HealthCall project to facilitate the transition to a 24 x 7 organization. The Technical Coordinator provided assistance in the development of the service level agreement, education of support staff, and the coordination of information systems departments and services needed to support the implementation of a new environment.

Implementation. The implementation of HealthCall required the coordination of member notification, employer group marketing, and provider education. The decision was made that HealthCall would be a standard component of the BCBSM and BCN local Michigan healthcare insurance products. This meant that 3.3 million members would be eligible for this service from day 1. Research shows that in call center implementations the initial call volumes are very high due to curiosity about the new service being offered. Therefore, one major problem that BCBSM faced was being positioned to respond to the initial call volumes to ensure long-term success of this service.

At first, it appeared that the membership could simply be divided into manageable volumes to load each month. When the issue was thoroughly examined, it became more complex.

Many of the BCBSM and BCN customers offer their employees several insurance products as well as options within those products. Therefore the employers did not want the service to be offered to only a few of their employees.

The BCNs needed to coordinate the roll-out of HealthCall with the education of their provider networks. The successful interaction with the PCP network was very important for overall member and provider satisfaction with the program.

The PCPs did not want to segment their practices so that a portion of their BCBSM/BCN practice had HealthCall, while others did not. The physicians wanted all or nothing with regard to their BCBSM/BCN patients covered by the HealthCall service.

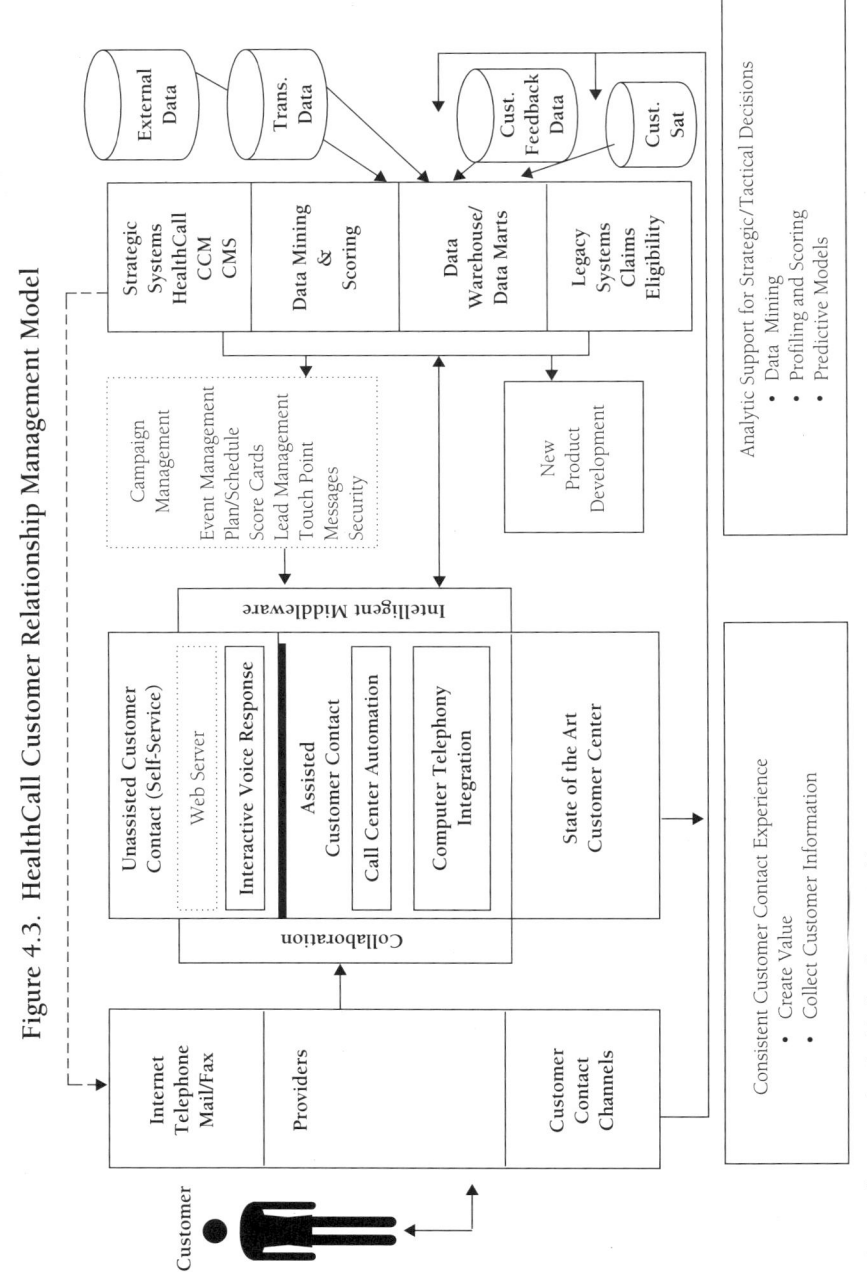

Figure 4.3. HealthCall Customer Relationship Management Model

Source: BlueCross BlueShield of Michigan. Used by permission.

This problem was resolved by using a blended approach to the implementation. For the BCBSM customers, employer groups were loaded into the system based on their renewal date. The implementation began on July 1, 1997, and was to end on June 1, 1998. The BCN members were added to the system in two segments, based on the BCN region to which the members belonged. The first segment was loaded on August 1, 1997, and the second on September 1, 1997. Within three months of implementation, HealthCall had over two million eligible members on the system.

Results

Currently, BCBSM has almost three million members enrolled in the HealthCall program. In the first six months of operation, the HealthCall program has worked with 16,000 callers whose healthcare questions ranged from croup to rashes to nausea to chest pain. In addition, the HealthCall system has had more than 23,000 calls to the audio health library.

To understand and assess the impact of HealthCall, BCBSM issued a HealthCall satisfaction survey to their HealthCall customers. This study found that:

- 82 percent of the callers are women.
- 82 percent of these callers are calling for themselves or for a child.
- 77 percent of the surveyed participants said that the HealthCall service improved the BCBSM image.
- 78 percent of the survey participants were satisfied with the services received.
- 88 percent of the survey participants were satisfied with HealthCall.
- 98 percent of the survey participants found the service easy to use.
- 90 percent of the survey participants indicated that they would use the HealthCall service again.

In addition, the survey also validated a change in healthcare consumer actions after using the HealthCall service.

- Before contacting HealthCall, 34 percent of the survey participants indicated that they intended to seek urgent care.
- After contacting HealthCall, 17 percent of the survey participants indicated that they intended to seek urgent care.

This represents a 50 percent decrease in patients seeking urgent care.

Based on the survey findings it was concluded that demand management does affect healthcare consumption in the following ways.

- It improves the healthcare consumer's overall satisfaction with the payer.
- It has a positive effect on the way BCBSM is viewed.
- It does change the healthcare consumers' medical choices.
- It allows healthcare consumers to make informed healthcare decisions.

The good news is that BCBSM healthcare consumers are using this service to obtain medical advice in determining the appropriate level of medical intervention. The service is growing and customers value it.

Conclusion

The healthcare consumer wants to make informed decisions related to his or her healthcare needs and/or purchases. To make an informed healthcare decision requires access to information. The healthcare consumer will use the information to make informed healthcare decisions if:

- The service is available.
- The information provided is helpful and easy to use.
- The service is delivered quickly and courteously.
- The service ensures confidentially.

BCBSM is making great strides in providing its membership with an integrated program that manages care by coordinating member health needs along the entire care continuum and providing a full spectrum of healthcare interventions.

The Future

The future for HealthCall offers many new opportunities to BCBSM and its customers.

- Linking the customer service systems to the Internet will allow more access to the BCBSM members for education, clinical reference material, and feedback on clinical episodes.
- Outbound campaigns can promote preventive health programs, support disease management programs, and inform customers of new services.
- Expanded integration with IHM programs will improve coordination of member services to provide a full spectrum of healthcare interventions

About the Authors

Mary Ann Baxter is a certified senior healthcare consultant with IBM.

Pamela S. Blankenship is the BCBSM Information Systems Manager responsible for the IHM project.

Edward Kornacki is a senior consultant and information technology architect with IBM's Global Services Practice.

Cathy McMahan works for IBM in the Healthcare Industry Consulting Practice.

Bill Epstein is a Consulting Information Systems Specialist (Certified) with IBM Global Services.

Call Centers in Healthcare: The Experience of One Health Maintenance Organization

Kathleen A. Christopherson, BSN, RN

Kaiser Permanente Foundation Health Plan of Texas is a group model health maintenance organization located in the Dallas–Ft. Worth Metroplex. Kaiser has been operating medical offices in this market for more than 15 years. Each of nine medical offices provides internal medicine, pediatric, and obstetric/gynecologic care to a membership of more than 130,000. Specialty services are provided in multiple locations. Medical advice by registered nurses using physician-written and -approved protocols is provided to our members around the clock.

Scheduling appointments and delivering medical advice can be a challenge when they are performed in each medical office. In 1995, Kaiser Permanente decided to establish a centralized call center to handle its functions of setting appointments and delivering medical advice. The Kaiser Call Center is located in Dallas and is easily reached from all parts of the Metroplex.

A centralized call center serves as a single, patient-friendly, 24-hour access point for Kaiser Permanente. The staff of the call center can help members understand their benefits as well as their rights and responsibilities. The creation of a single access center merges the functions of setting appointments, providing physician-directed medical advice, an answering service, and switchboard operations for the company.

Because each medical office was scheduling its own appointments and had its own medical advice processes, a major reengineering effort was required before the opening of the call center. Appointment agents and nurses were offered the opportunity to transfer their work to the call center location and most accepted that transfer.

The Kaiser Call Center was built with an eye toward an ergonomically appropriate and aesthetically pleasing environment. Also of prime consideration was the ability to physically interact with one's coworkers. CenterCore workstations were selected with positions for five operators. The positions of the workstation pods in the call center allow interaction among coworkers while the sound-absorbent partitions minimize the ambient noise in the department.

The heart of the workstation pod contains an air filtration system for reducing viruses, allergens, and dust. The air filtration system has significantly reduced the spread of illnesses in this 7000–square-foot open space room. Three "cold and flu seasons" have come and gone since the opening of the call center. Absence due to communicable illness has been less than 2 percent of the total workforce during the peak of cold and flu season.

Ergonomically designed chairs were selected with hydraulic controls for optimum positioning by each operator. Manipulating keyboards with wrist supports reduces the cumulative trauma from repetitive typing. Foot rests were provided to reduce the stress placed on the lower back when sitting for long periods.

Each agent and nurse has a personal computer and an automated call distributor (ACD) phone. All operators are required to use a headset with the phone. Being part of a large, integrated healthcare system has allowed the call center to provide its staff with educational programs presented by licensed physical therapists to further lessen the potential for physical discomfort.

With centralization came the need to accurately predict call volumes and then schedule the appropriate number of people to handle the volume. Software was purchased to interface with the Meridian Max switch and forecast our staffing needs. Initially, historical data from each medical office were loaded into the system and initial staffing levels forecasted. Each day of operation brings more accuracy to this system. Accurate staffing is now possible, which leads to a high level of service to members and an equally high level of productivity from agents and nurses.

Since all of Kaiser's appointment setting functions and clinical information systems reside on the local area network, bringing this functionality into the call center was a simple process. We very quickly learned, however, that the memory requirements were significantly increased in the call center personal computers to run multiple applications at the same time. During our two years of operation, additional applications have been written for use in the call center. We have seen our needs grow from 486 systems to a Windows NT environment.

The primary objective in using a centralized call center approach was to dramatically improve customer service to our members. Before the advent of the call center, call volumes varied widely in each medical office, leading to long hold times in some areas and short times in others. Centralization allowed a smoothing out of the peaks and valleys in volumes, and we now provide an average answer speed of 30 seconds or less. Additional advantages were seen in an overall reduction in the number of staff members required to meet the demand. This has allowed a more efficient distribution of staff throughout the organization. Another advantage has been the fact that the member can call one number and have all his or her needs met. If the service requested is not supported by the call center, the member can be easily and quickly transferred to the appropriate person. Members only have to remember one number to call to get what they need.

Centralized appointment setting allows more creativity and flexibility when meeting the needs of members. In 1997 Kaiser's department of preventive health services began looking at making mammography more accessible. In late April 1997, a program called "Self-Referred Mammography" was begun. Women meeting a few basic criteria, i.e., 40 years or older and absence of clinical signs of breast problems, were encouraged to obtain a screening mammogram. The call center was ideal for offering this service. Each woman who met the criteria and called the call center to make an appointment for an annual physical examination was offered the opportunity to schedule her mammogram at the same time. Women who met the criteria and called to schedule other appointments were given the same opportunity. We compared the numbers of screening mammograms completed during the same eight–month time frame in 1996 and 1997. In 1996, before self-referral mammography was possible, 4194 screening mammograms were completed. In 1997, the number of completed screening mammograms rose to 8005 (Figure 5.1). The control afforded by centralization of staff has shown a remarkable improvement in this process.

One of the challenges facing healthcare providers is how to reduce the number of appointments wasted due to patients' failure to appear for the

Figure 5.1. Comparison of Mammography Rates Before (1996) and After (1997) Implementation of the Self-Referral Mammography Program

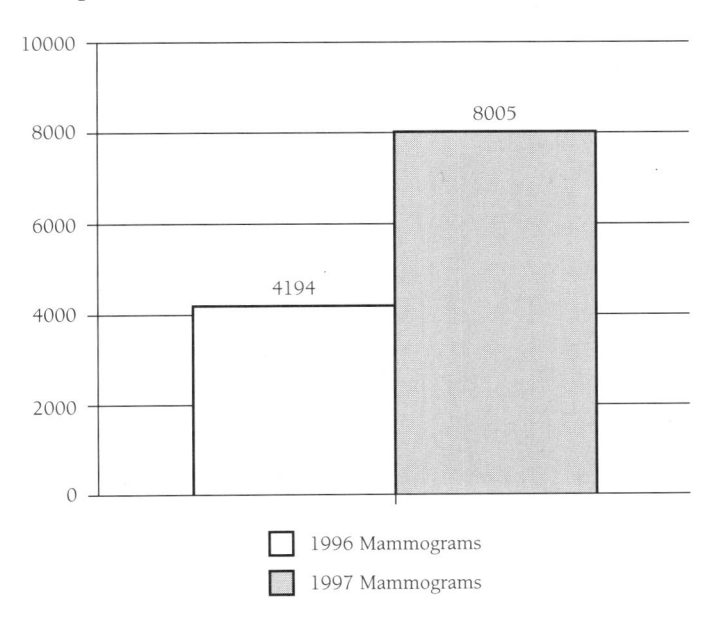

appointment, commonly known as "no-shows." A centralized call center presents the opportunity to make confirmation calls without affecting the productivity of the office staff. Even with perfect staffing forecasting, there are times of low call volume in the call center when our appointment agents simply wait for an in-coming call. During these periods of down-time, our appointment agents confirm a list of appointments for each healthcare provider. The measure of success of the confirmation call program is the rather dramatic reduction in our no-show rate calculated during the same three–month time period in 1996 and 1997 (Figure 5.2).

The vision of Kaiser Permanente is to provide superior healthcare at an affordable cost in a manner that pleases its members. Centralization of appointment scheduling and medical advice processes has constituted an extensive quality assurance program which quickly identifies any training needs. Our members can be assured of accurate and timely responses to their needs from the call center. Member satisfaction with the appointment scheduling and medical advice processes have steadily climbed in our two-year history and is now at a 99 percent level of high satisfaction.

Frequently, members need help deciding what the best course of action is for them. Our call center provides continuous medical advice by registered nurses using physician-written and-approved protocols. This advice can range from what immunizations are required and when, to what to do during a life-threatening emergency. Many members simply want to be able to confer with a healthcare professional to be sure that they are on the right track. It is enormously comforting for parents to be able to speak with a registered nurse who

Figure 5.2. Comparison of No-Show Rates Before (1996) and After (1997) Implementation of the Appointment Confirmation Call Program

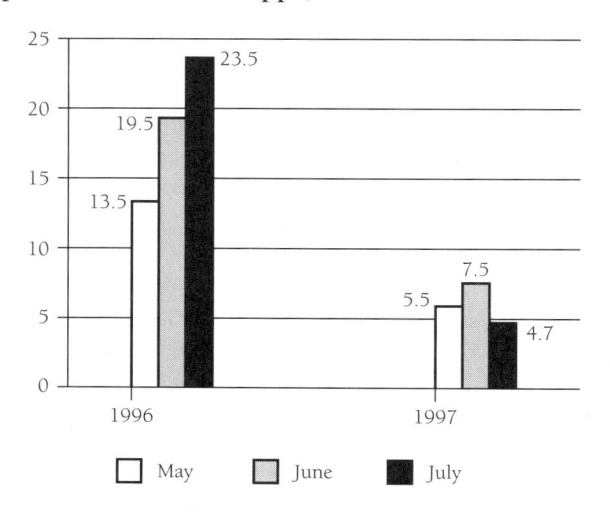

Month	1996	1997
May	13.5	5.5
June	19.5	7.5
July	23.5	4.7

knows what their pediatrician recommends. When that service can be provided in the middle of the night, as can be done in the call center, the member not only is comforted but also uses the appropriate level of care. Middle of the night trips to the emergency room, while sometimes necessary, can often be avoided with appropriate medical advice.

"Demand management," a current industry buzzword, can be provided in a centralized call center. Our medical advice nurses use physician-written protocols to help members make the best decision on what level of care is necessary. Many minor injuries and illnesses, e.g., cold and flu symptoms, allergies, and symptoms of upper respiratory infections, can be handled at home with medical advice. Members can be called a few days after the medical advice intervention to assess the success of, and satisfaction with, the process. When a trip to the medical office or the emergency department is appropriate, the medical advice nurses can schedule an appointment or facilitate the trip to the emergency department. Early notification of the emergency department by the medical advice nurse smooths the process for the member.

Advantages to physicians are seen in the "first-call triage" function of medical advice. All calls for medical advice come to the registered nurses. Physicians are called by the nurse who can provide a professional assessment of the situation. The nurse can provide the physician with current laboratory and radiology results for the patient as well as prior history of illness and medication utilization. This service is of particular importance after the offices have closed. A centralized call center is ideal for providing this service to the physician at all times of the day and night.

Initial reactions by the clinicians to the call center concept were not always positive. Centralized appointment scheduling can be seen as a loss of control. Maintaining good relationships between the call center and our clinicians continues to be a top priority. Critical to the success of the program is attendance by call center supervisors at medical office meetings. Face-to-face interaction solves many concerns. We installed a supervisor hotline in the call center for immediate access to a supervisor. This portable phone is carried with the supervisor on duty at all times. This occasionally leads to some interesting background noise but has been extremely successful in maintaining relationships.

The Kaiser Call Center has been able to provide excellent customer service to its members and clinicians with technology that allows its staff to be efficient, accurate, and knowledgeable. We have been able to establish a safe and pleasing work environment for more than 100 people and look forward to our future growth.

About the Author

Kathleen A. Christopherson, BSN, RN, is the Administrator of the Southwest Division Call Center for Kaiser Permanente.

How Technology Can Make You a Hero with Your Customers

Dick Herrmann; Mary Bryant

With all the advances made by our country on the clinical side of healthcare, the administrative side of the industry remains virtually without significant automation. Today it is the norm for financial institutions to offer their customers various methods of automated banking, trading, etc., using interactive voice response (IVR), computer telephony integration (CTI), Internet applications, and integrated IVR/Internet solutions. This same technology can be applied to healthcare administration.

Effective healthcare automation solutions are designed to benefit a varied audience within the healthcare administration industry. There are products or services of interest to third-party administrators, plan providers, and major employers with in-house benefits administration.

Examples of automated healthcare solutions include benefits enrollment, claim status, and eligibility. The major benefits of automating these functions include data accuracy, convenience, and time and cost savings.

Healthcare administration firms devote significant portions of their operating budgets to establishing and maintaining call centers. Yet without proper integration of data and accessible links to customers, call center productivity cannot be fully realized. More and more customers today want greater freedom to access their information when they want and need it. You can turn this need for self-service into savings for your company.

Each of the automation solutions mentioned has the potential to significantly affect the productivity of a call center. The key is to design and deploy an effective automation solution that meets your internal needs and those of your customers. Lack of automation of these functions can be a tremendous drain on expensive, highly trained knowledge resources. On the other hand, call centers that use automation techniques for each of these functions enjoy higher productivity by their service staff, increased customer satisfaction, and higher service staff morale because the large majority of routine inquiries are now handled without human intervention. This leaves service staff free to handle the more challenging situations requiring their expertise. Thus service representatives are more content and call center resources are more effectively used.

Call centers are not the only winners in the automation game. Employers and employees also enjoy benefits. By automating plan provider/administrator functions, employers and their employees gain greater access to their data. They can now access their information 24 hours per day, seven days a week. That results in fewer calls to the employer benefits department and more satisfied employees with respect to benefits administration. In the case of benefits enrollment, employees and employers alike can have immediate confirmation that the enrollment transaction has been completed. In addition, they can easily receive timely written confirmation of their enrollment elections via mail, fax, or even e-mail wherever available.

Another major benefit for all parties is the availability of reporting options. Whether you are the plan provider/administrator or the employer, timely and accurate reporting is critical to effectively managing your business. An effective call center automation solution for healthcare must include a timely reporting function. Your customers *want* information, and they want it quickly. The more information to which your customers have convenient access, the fewer inquiries your call center will receive.

Why Should You Automate?

Customer satisfaction, lower operating costs, product differentiation, faster service, and accurate data and reporting are just a few of the benefits. In this article, we will focus on the advantages of automating the benefits enrollment process. One of the most labor-intensive activities in which a healthcare administration provider participates each year is open enrollment. Begin the transformation from carrier to "hero" by eliminating the source of the problem for and your customer and you: *paperwork*. Paperwork seems like a necessary evil when it comes to benefits enrollment. Year after year it is the same process for enrollment. After all, "it has always been done this way." If you are the health insurance provider, for example, you only have one set of forms to contend with each year, but your customer is faced with the enrollment process for medical, dental, vision, Section 125 savings plans, and so forth. It all starts around September 1, and goes well into the beginning of the new year, ending hopefully sometime in February. During this period, we appear to lose all perspective on our real mission in the healthcare industry because we are drowning in paperwork and the time delays created by the processing of paperwork (Figure 6.1).

You are all too familiar with open enrollment. Your client services team is fielding those tense telephone calls and tap dancing in status meetings with clients.

"Who's enrolled so far?"

"What plan has a higher participation rate this year—health maintenance organization (HMO) or preferred provider organization?"

"It's a positive enrollment. Everybody has to turn in a form. Do you have Sally Smith's form yet? We sent it last week."

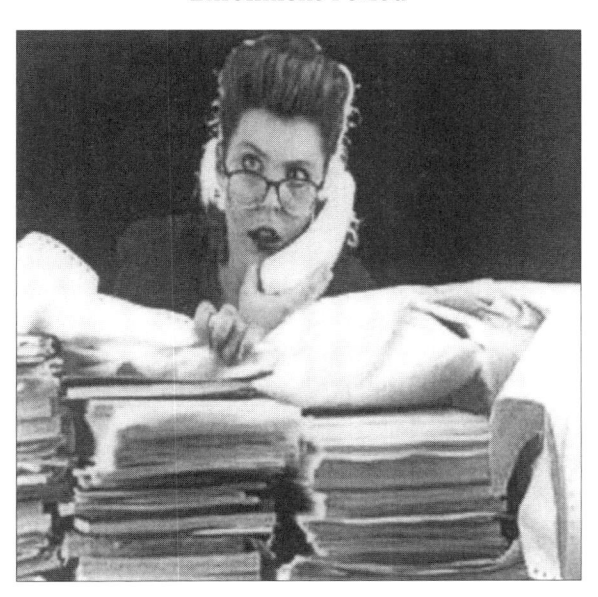

Figure 6.1. Processing of Paperwork During an Open Enrollment Period

It does not have to be this way. You can change your situation without taking on a second full-time job as a voice response unit (VRU) programmer or Internet Web master. Your client services staff will love you, your management will be delighted, your customers will be shocked, your staff will be thrilled, and you will once again have time to focus on your core functions.

You already have a big piece of the puzzle in place—your call center. But are you satisfied with the efficiency of your call center? Even more importantly, are your customers satisfied with the efficiency and effectiveness of your call center? If the answer to either of these questions is less than a resounding yes, it may be time to take inventory of how you use this very important tool. Make your call center work proactively for you and your customers. With proper planning and the right automation solution, you can enhance your call center with IVR and Internet technology to tackle the open enrollment paperwork problem. Remember that the paper is a problem not only for you. It is a significant problem for your customers too.

Employee benefits managers are beginning to ask these tough questions when it comes to enrollment.

"Why doesn't it change?"

"Why haven't my vendors bothered to change with the technology?"

"Don't they appreciate the amount of time we have to spend sending out forms, checking and rechecking to make sure all areas are correct?"

In fact, more and more employers are making automated enrollment an issue in their initial contracts and renewal negotiations. Why the sudden interest from the employer perspective? The benefits of process reengineering have finally reached the last bastion of the paper dynasties, human resources (HR) and benefits departments! If your customers are demanding automation and you cannot offer a solution, start investigating your options now. If you do not, somebody will do it. More and more insurers and third-party administrators are beginning to automate their enrollment process. Your customers may go to a vendor down the street and get exactly what they want and need. With the following components, you can solve the paperwork problems for your customers and yourself with the same solution:

- An automated process that allows easy access for employees, the HR/benefits department, and the provider's enrollment customer service staff
- A system that lets employees enter personal choices quickly and easily
- A system that is convenient
- A system that does not require a costly equipment investment
- A system that monitors enrollment progress on a dynamic basis
- An intelligent system that prevents the input of erroneous data
- A system that produces up-to-the-minute reports
- A system that quickly confirms, in writing, employee enrollment choices
- A system that allows customers access whenever they need it

Does this sound too good to be true? Well, it really is not. Today's technology will easily handle such an operation. The trick is to find professionals who understand benefits and provider organizations and have a commanding knowledge of the technology required to design the system.

How do we know it works? Let us examine the case study of an HR manager who knew exactly what she wanted and the resulting automation solution provided by her very responsive carrier.

Kathy Buehner, HR Manager for the City of Arlington, Texas, was faced with mounds of paperwork and an already heavily tasked team of employees in her department. The thought of one more open enrollment paperwork frenzy was not acceptable to her. So she made automated enrollment a condition of her renewal with her long-time health insurance carrier. She did not want to leave her insurance carrier, with whom she had long enjoyed a successful relationship, but she wanted to begin the move to a paperless environment. The carrier valued the relationship too. They did not want to lose her business, but they did not have an automated solution. So they got busy and did their homework on what type of solution would best serve their long-time client.

After much research, they settled on a fully integrated call center approach. They could have just put together a simple VRU application that handled the easy part of enrollment like "I want everything the same as last year, no new dependents, etc." That would have been good, but what about all the employees who do need to add dependents? After all, open enrollment is just that—"open." That is the one time during the year when employees can add and delete dependents with few restrictions. No, Kathy needed a full-service application. She needed an application that would allow her employees to make almost every type of enrollment change through some sort of automation. So the final application was born out of that lofty goal: "to accommodate my employees' enrollment needs." That is just what her carrier did. The following is a summary of the system.

A voice response application was designed to handle the basic enrollment functions for each plan. Based on Kathy's requirements, enrollment for her medical, dental, life, and Section 125 plans were to be automated by her health insurance carrier. The eligibility requirements and major exceptions were programmed into the application to ensure that employees not eligible for an HMO, for example, were not allowed to enroll in such a plan. Each plan's rules were accounted for in the application. It was clearly observed in the design process that certain situations were not easily handled simply by using a voice response application, but would require assistance from a customer service representative. The question was, "Whose customer service representative?" For example, adding a dependent by spelling the name over a telephone keypad is not user-friendly in the least. It is best handled over the Internet or by some sort of human intervention. Well, Kathy was not ready to jump to Internet access at the employee level. She was concerned about the lack of personal computers and Internet access among her employee population. But what could be done about adding employees? She did not want any part of a paper process. That would defeat her whole purpose.

Once again, her carrier rose to the occasion. Why not integrate the voice response application into their existing call center so that they could handle the calls that required assistance? They had well-trained employees ready to answer calls, but how could their call center representatives get access to the data from the voice response application? Their thorough research in the beginning paid off well because the consulting firm they engaged had the solution they needed. They were able to use a secure Web-enabled application to access the same database accessed by the voice response application. As a result, enrollees who wanted assistance with their enrollment could transfer out to a fully trained customer service representative equipped with all the information needed to complete the enrollment. This is significant from a data processing standpoint as well. Regardless of whether the customer service representative or the enrollee made the change, it was recorded in the same database. This ensures the synchronization of data between the carrier and the employer.

As is usually the case with employee benefits administration, to every rule there is an exception. Kathy and her staff needed online access to the enrollment process from their offices. There may be times when they need to override an enrollment condition or actually enroll an employee who needed a little extra assistance. Kathy's carrier arranged for her to have online access to the same Internet-based browser application that was being used in their call center. Now Kathy had instantaneous access to all her enrollment records.

The last piece of the puzzle was a written confirmation sent to employees' home addresses which summarized and confirmed their enrollment elections for the coming year. This confirmation served as written notice of the employees' elections and reassured employees that their enrollment elections were actually recorded.

Kathy benefited in various ways. She successfully eliminated the paperwork from her enrollment process. There were no forms for the payroll department to input, no forms for the administrative staff to file, no forms to be collected and bundled for distribution to the carrier, and lastly, no cries from employees that they really had sent in their form and that it must have been lost in the mail. Not only did she eliminate paper from her process, but also she replaced the paper with *information.* That was what she wanted in the first place, and the paper served as her only readily available source until now. As future open enrollment sessions draw to a close, Kathy has her finger on the pulse of the entire enrollment process. She knows who is enrolling in what plan, who is not capitalizing on the life insurance benefits available to them, and who is participating in the Section 125 plans. With information available to her throughout the enrollment process, Kathy can afford to focus her energies on really educating employees on the benefits package and helping them take full advantage of what is available to them. From Kathy's point of view, that is what it is all about. She adds, "My goal for several years has been to increase productivity and reduce costs by automating and outsourcing as many functions as possible so that my staff can concentrate on customer service. Open enrollment is one of the most obvious places to start." Her carrier also benefited in many ways, not the least of which was her satisfaction as a long-time customer.

Data Verification

One of the biggest headaches associated with the standard methods used for processing enrollment data (other than the sheer volume of information to be entered) is the redundancy of data input between employer HR systems and carriers and the associated error and data mismatches. The more the data is manually handled the greater the likelihood of errors such as transposition and omission of data. A properly automated enrollment system with "edits" for data verification and completion will greatly alleviate this problem. The end result of an open enrollment session can be dates of birth consistent across databases; spelling of names consistent across databases; and enrollment records complete with names, social security numbers, correct address information, correct dependent information, and validated primary care physician designations where required. Again, if you design an effective solution that coordinates data between carrier and employer, your resulting data can be completely cleansed and shared with all parties. That is a benefit for everyone. When was the last time your enrollment data actually matched?

Timeliness of Information

Gone are the days of scrambling to process those enrollment forms that straggle in just before the information technology job is due to run. Gone are the days of not knowing how many enrollments are not yet accounted for in positive enrollment situations. Gone are the days of having to apologize for keying in the wrong data for the wrong enrollee! The days of loading the enrollment job once and populating the system with clean data are here!

Evaluating Automated Enrollment Solutions

What should you consider when evaluating the move to automated enrollment solutions?

Define Your Goals. First you should define what you want to accomplish. Automated enrollment is a broad term.

- Do you want to provide enrollment services for your product only?
- Do you want to provide enrollment services for all of your customers' benefit plans?
- Should the system give enrollees the choice of enrolling over the telephone or the Internet or both? (Consider offering both access media because it eliminates trying to poll who has Internet access and who does not. It really does not matter anyway. Let the enrollee make the choice of which access method to use.)
- What level of transaction tracking do you want?
- Do you wish to have access to online reporting for your customers and yourself?
- Do you want your enrollment specialists to be able to enter enrollment data?
- Do you want your customers' benefits department employees to be able to enter enrollment data?
- Do you want to integrate the VRU and/or Web application with your existing call center for a higher level of customer service?
- Who will create enrollment training documents and forms (critical to the success of any automated program)?

Remember to think about all the tasks that you want to eliminate, and it will be easy to define your goals!

Do It Myself or Hire Someone? You must evaluate whether you want to create the system yourself or have someone do it for you. This comes down to a simple question. What is your primary role? If it is not system development, then outsource this as quickly as possible. Look for someone who will provide the services that you are requesting in the time frame that you require. However, be cautious. Someone who claims that it can be done in 30 days probably is not telling you the whole story or does not understand your needs with regard to an integrated automated enrollment system.

Evaluate Your Budget Constraints. Systems should not require a great deal of up-front expense; some systems are available through service bureaus. Most service bureaus will price the system and services on either a transaction basis or a per-employee per-month basis. The latter spreads your expense across 12 months, which may be better for your existing budget.

Do not forget to do a cost justification. The flowchart in Figure 6.2 can be used to illustrate the costs associated with the standard manual enrollment process from the perspective of both the employer and the carrier. Take the time to complete the flowchart exercise. Be sure to get input from all the departments involved with open enrollment processing. If your company can save hundreds of precious hours during enrollment months, show management the benefits!

If your existing staff does not include a programmer with experience on one of the various VRU platforms and you want to make this an in-house function, you can hire someone with this experience or get one of your existing staff members trained on one of the various platforms.

Your Internet needs will be as follows:

- A developer(s) proficient in real world use of hypertext markup language (HTML), Java, JavaScript, active server pages (ASP), structured query language (SQL), graphics production, etc.
- A system administrator(s) who can manage network security, performance tuning, and hardware and software maintenance.
- Ideally a Web master for this type of project who also has the skills to tie in the Web application to the IVR.

For an in-house solution, you will also need the following equipment in addition to the appropriate staff. For voice response solutions only:

- Network services for a toll-free telephone number
- Sufficient port capacity within your telephone switch to handle peak call traffic
- Sufficient VRU port capacity to handle peak call traffic
- A database server with appropriate processor speed and storage capacity that is compatible with your VRU platform software
- Redundant VRU platforms for disaster recovery

How Technology Can Make You a Hero with Your Customers 67

Figure 6.2. Flowchart Illustrating the Costs (in Dollars and Days) Associated with the Standard Manual Enrollment Process

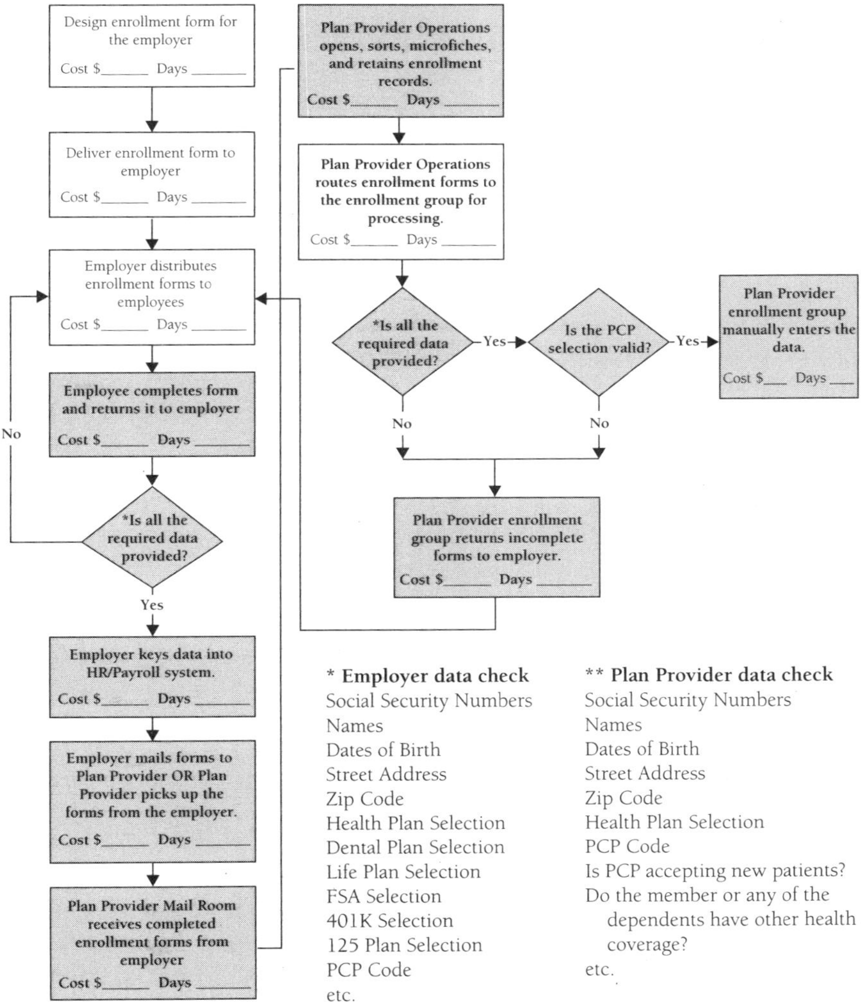

```
┌─────────────────────────┐        ┌─────────────────────────────┐
│ Design enrollment form  │        │ Plan Provider Operations    │
│ for the employer        │        │ opens, sorts, microfiches,  │
│ Cost $____ Days ____    │        │ and retains enrollment      │
└───────────┬─────────────┘        │ records.                    │
            │                       │ Cost $____ Days ____        │
            ▼                       └──────────────┬──────────────┘
┌─────────────────────────┐                        │
│ Deliver enrollment form │                        ▼
│ to employer             │        ┌─────────────────────────────┐
│ Cost $____ Days ____    │        │ Plan Provider Operations    │
└───────────┬─────────────┘        │ routes enrollment forms to  │
            │                      │ the enrollment group for    │
            ▼                      │ processing.                 │
┌─────────────────────────┐        │ Cost $____ Days ____        │
│ Employer distributes    │        └──────────────┬──────────────┘
│ enrollment forms to     │◄──┐                   │
│ employees               │   │                   ▼
│ Cost $____ Days ____    │   │       ◇*Is all the◇ ──Yes──► ◇Is the PCP◇ ──Yes──► ┌───────────────────┐
└───────────┬─────────────┘   │        required data            selection valid?    │ Plan Provider     │
            │                 │        provided?                                    │ enrollment group  │
            ▼                 │          │                        │                  │ manually enters   │
┌─────────────────────────┐   │          No                       No                 │ the data.         │
│ Employee completes form │   │          │                        │                  │ Cost $__ Days __  │
│ and returns it to       │   │          ▼                        ▼                  └───────────────────┘
│ employer                │   │   ┌──────────────────────────────────┐
│ Cost $____ Days ____    │   │   │ Plan Provider enrollment group   │
└───────────┬─────────────┘   │   │ returns incomplete forms to      │
     No     │                 │   │ employer.                        │
  ◄─────────┤                 │   │ Cost $____ Days ____             │
            ▼                 │   └──────────────────────────────────┘
       ◇*Is all the◇          │
        required data         │
        provided?             │
            │                 │
           Yes                │
            ▼                 │
┌─────────────────────────┐   │
│ Employer keys data into │   │
│ HR/Payroll system.      │   │
│ Cost $____ Days ____    │   │
└───────────┬─────────────┘   │
            ▼                 │
┌─────────────────────────┐   │
│ Employer mails forms to │   │
│ Plan Provider OR Plan   │   │
│ Provider picks up the   │   │
│ forms from the employer.│   │
│ Cost $____ Days ____    │   │
└───────────┬─────────────┘   │
            ▼                 │
┌─────────────────────────┐   │
│ Plan Provider Mail Room │   │
│ receives completed      │   │
│ enrollment forms from   │───┘
│ employer                │
│ Cost $____ Days ____    │
└─────────────────────────┘
```

* Employer data check
Social Security Numbers
Names
Dates of Birth
Street Address
Zip Code
Health Plan Selection
Dental Plan Selection
Life Plan Selection
FSA Selection
401K Selection
125 Plan Selection
PCP Code
etc.

** Plan Provider data check
Social Security Numbers
Names
Dates of Birth
Street Address
Zip Code
Health Plan Selection
PCP Code
Is PCP accepting new patients?
Do the member or any of the
    dependents have other health
    coverage?
etc.

Source: The Interactive Information Institute, Inc. Used by permission.

For IVR and Internet solutions, all of the above plus:

- A permanent, high-speed connection to the Internet (T1)
- A network of servers in an installation that provides a secure, fault-tolerant architecture (data and hardware)
- High-capacity, high-performance servers
- At least one Web server (dedicated)
- At least one database server (dedicated) with a modern relational database management system (RDBMS)
- A firewall and security policies to prevent tampering
- A stable development environment with version control

On the other hand, you may choose to completely outsource this functionality. There are consulting companies and service bureaus with platforms that can be used for your enrollment programs. These firms typically perform all the programming, project management, back-office processing, customer support, and disaster recovery services required for an enrollment project. The service bureau will need to design custom application software for your particular benefit program. In most cases, this can be done with 90 to 120 days' notice. Make sure the service provider has the right type of equipment to guarantee high-grade service. That is, when employees call in or connect via the Internet, they do not get busy signals. Look for an experienced management team and check its references. Be aware that this type of technology for integrated telephony and Internet services is new, that is, within the last couple of years. So, beware of claims of having done this for years and years. It just isn't so!

Your customer will need very little equipment to support an integrated enrollment solution. The equipment required of your customer is simply a telephone and a computer with Internet access. Almost every employee has access to one or the other.

As discussed, there are many ways to automate your call center to improve its efficiency and effectiveness. We have looked at one very time-consuming manual process that can easily be automated to better serve your needs and those of your customers, but enrollment is just one of many examples. Whatever section of the healthcare industry you represent, you have processes and customers who can benefit from automated solutions. Examine the calls your customer service representatives receive on a daily basis. Identify the calls that involve routine inquiries. Such calls are excellent candidates for automation. Remember that effective automation techniques serve as an enhancement to your service, not a replacement.

If your customers are not yet asking for automation solutions, it will not be long before they start. So stop shuffling paperwork for four months a year and free yourself to do the things you were hired to do in the first place. Also have some fun along the way. Implementing an automated enrollment program is going to make you a hero!

About the Authors

Dick Herrmann is President and Chief Executive Officer of The Interactive Information Institute, TI 3, Inc., Dallas, Texas (www.ti3.com).

Mary Bryant is Director of Healthcare Services for The Interactive Information Institute, TI 3, Inc.

Creating a Vision for Your Medical Call Center

Julie L. Barr; Sue Laufenberg; Brian L. Sieckman

Introduction

Managed care is a driving force in much of the change occurring in the healthcare industry. One of those changes is the adoption of medical call center (MCC) technologies. Simply put, an MCC conducts a triage of the patient using the least costly, medically appropriate level of care. Cost savings, along with patient care, are the key managed care yardsticks of today's provider organizations.

An MCC supports an organization's mission by helping deliver services in a timely, cost-effective, and patient-acceptable manner. An MCC consolidates fragmented requests for physician referral, health guidance, and hospital information. It provides a one-call, central access point over the telephone or the Internet. An MCC is a repository of help and information, strengthening customers relationships and increasing referrals.

The MCC also documents dollars captured in fee-for-service systems and dollars saved in managed care systems. An MCC has proven financial benefits; studies have shown that for every $1 invested in this technology, $4.75 is saved through better selection and use of available services. Besides decreasing medical costs, MCCs can provide many other personal health management functions including the following.

- Increased medical compliance
- Chronic disease management
- Behavior changes monitoring
- Self-assessment measures
- Self-help and goal management
- Medical news and information
- Provider-patient communications
- Gateway to physicians, pharmacists, counselors, and other caregivers
- Nurse triage support

- Physician referrals
- Demographic updates, insurance claim submission, and follow-up
- Interactive voice response (IVR) services (i.e., prescription refill, patient satisfaction surveys)
- Public relations, education, and marketing information
- Medical telemetry/telemedicine connections

Call centers, coupled with other approaches to patient education, have evolved into what is called "personal healthcare management," an important way for managed care entities to reduce the cost of covering lives while maintaining or improving quality of care. Personal health management programs, an umbrella term that includes MCCs as a key component, covered about 8 million lives in the United States in 1994. Currently, call centers respond to almost 100 million calls per year and cover about 35 million lives (with virtually no incidence of litigation). At this rate, by the year 2000, MCCs could cover 100 million lives.

As patients continue to be more proactive in their desire for information and participation in medical care decisions, providers will need to leverage all the technology available to them. The MCC is one tool that allows organizations to increase patient access, involvement, and satisfaction through service customized to each patient's needs.

MCCs are not typical of the information systems projects undertaken by many provider organizations. However, the savvy chief executive officer, chief information officer, or chief operating officer will easily see them as a vehicle for successfully implementing competitive marketplace strategies. Ideally, the management team will have a solid business plan and organizational mission on which to base tactical executions such as MCCs. In fact, the MCC platform can achieve multiple objectives by integrating existing applications. To define your own call center vision, the following must be kept in mind.

- How can the MCC become the physician office of the future?
- What features, functions, and applications are currently available for MCCs?
- What level of service does your organization want to provide?
- What is your vision?
- How does the MCC fit your organization's strategic planning process?
- Should you outsource MCC services or build your own system?
- How do you gain internal support to sell your idea to your organization?

MCCs of the Future

All of the MCC technology solutions described herein exist today. However, the challenges for a provider organization are far greater than technology. As with any purchase, the decision-maker wants to be certain that it is the "best buy for the money" and that it can leverage existing investments through integration.

Creating a Vision for Your Medical Call Center

Imagine primary care providers (PCPs) and specialists only seeing patients in their office when it is absolutely necessary, with nurse and patient monitoring being conducted the rest of the time from the "electronic physician office," the call center. Imagine being able to reach a patient any time, anywhere, through any selected communication device (telephone, pager, Internet, voice mail, fax, etc.). Imagine the PCP having care protocols available at his or her fingertips; and that is not all, wellness information, recent medical research, health assessments, nutritional information, and healthy goal setting with patient input are all possible. Imagine the potential for early detection and diagnosis of disease through frequent and meaningful patient intervention. Imagine creating a technology platform for delivering disease management solutions directly to the individual patient and then allowing for related patient-provider interactions. Now, also imagine fingertip access to complete patient record information; patient risk assessment information; patient nutritional plans; patient exercise goals; immediate, interactive access to a patient's case workers; disease-specific medical research for PCP and patient; interactive patient access any time to care provider (nurse or other clinician); patient satisfaction surveys; disease management outcomes; behavioral change management; moving beyond demand and disease management to customized health; and more.

Each technology discussed here brings distinct functions and benefits to the call center. Internet capabilities allow patients to communicate with the caregiver over the Internet. These can be in a store-and-forward mode or they can be real-time transmissions. They also can be further integrated with several other communication technologies to create a multitiered communication process, using, for example, a combination of paging, fax, voice mail, and e-mail. Figure 7.1 depicts the capability to expand the MCC into a true care center. The reality is that all of this will become standard in the MCCs of the future, but the underlying technologies are here today! Dictating when specific technologies are deployed are factors such as whether a business plan has been written which includes the vision, mission, timeline, and competitive assessment; whether the budget has been allocated, not just planned; and stratification of the patient population that will be served by the MCC (e.g., bed-ridden chronically ill, ambulatory chronically ill, homebound chronically ill, etc.).

Trends in the MCC Environment

MCCs currently provide customer service information and triage services within the community at large or for specific patients under a managed health plan. Nearly all of their responses are to inbound and patient-initiated inquiries . As patients continue to have more say in their healthcare decisions, the MCC can become an ever increasingly important strategic initiative for the healthcare provider. Consider the following market facts.

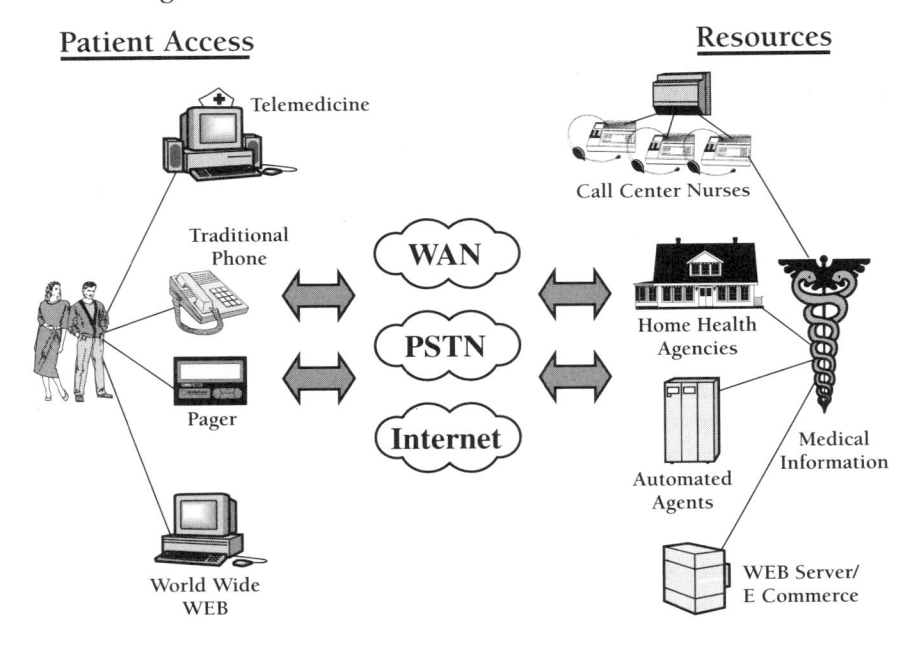

Figure 7.1. Patient/Professional Access to Information

- Patients will continue to drive the demand for access to high-quality information regarding their health.
- Studies continue to suggest that 40 percent to 80 percent of all patients entering the healthcare system do not need a physician's care.
- A recent survey found that 77 percent of patients would give up a personal visit with their PCP if they could get credible, fast information on the Internet or over the telephone.

These findings lead us to believe that, although MCCs will still be used for nurse triage or demand management services, there will be an evolution toward providing personalized healthcare or disease management plans. Healthcare organizations will begin to conduct health risk assessment services, leading to patient stratification according to individual need for level of care and intervention. Patients' preferences for receiving information and their ability to assimilate that information will also be calculated. This leads to a personal health management plan that can be fully developed and delivered through the MCC.

Technology trends will result in more deployment of outbound, predictive dialing capabilities in the call center to deliver care plans to patients. Integrating Internet and Web technology will allow the center to create personalized Web sites for their patients. Intelligent routing for knowledge worker applications will speed patient access to the appropriate nurse/agent, in turn increasing the use of decision-making technologies like decision support, patient information, and practice guidelines. IVR will become increasingly important as additional patient service applications, such as drug interaction information and audio text health libraries, are developed.

According to a 1998 series of focus groups conducted by Sprint Healthcare Systems, providers will continue to search for solutions that increase efficiencies and productivity for their organizations. They will look for technologies with which they have experience and which can be easily integrated into their current environment. Finally, vendors must be able to work closely with customers to devise solid cost/benefit analyses of any new equipment.

Implementation and deployment methods of MCC services will continue to be mixed. In 1998–1999, it is believed that 50 percent to 60 percent of early adopters will select a service bureau option. By 1999–2000, the trend will shift to in-house systems due to increased economies of scale and matured learning curves of providers.

MCC Categories

MCCs can be divided into two categories based on their functions: administrative (or operator services) and clinical (nurse triage, wellness, and medical counseling). Healthcare organizations can place these functions either in a common site or divide the locations by functionality.

An administrative or operator services call center is designed for seamless integration of existing telephone, paging and alarm systems, providing screen pops, screen dialing, and intelligent call handling. Applications can include directory services, on-call calendars, answering services, paging, physician registry, and administrative reporting. The system is driven from an intelligent personal computer workstation providing screen-based interactive call processing and directory functions. Interactive call processing functions include automatic screen display of incoming calls, call transfers, conferencing, speed dialing, message waiting activation, and other private branch exchange (PBX) console-type operations. As the healthcare industry continues to merge and consolidate, creating a seamless entry point for patients becomes essential to patient satisfaction with quality.

A nurse triage call center is the most widely used type of MCC today. Using automated guidelines and a series of algorithms to determine appropriate level of care, the nurse triage center can determine the patient's needs or respond to a question for self care. As managed care and capitation continue to pressure expenses, demand management or more appropriate care management tools will continue to evolve. This inbound service can save the organization patient costs through proper patient triage. However, such a center continues to be a high-cost item for the healthcare provider; providers need to learn how to generate revenues from them.

A wellness MCC can be designed to provide patients, employees, and professional staff with health information services. By adding voice mail and IVR systems to the center, both administrative and clinical applications can be offered. Applications such as benefits enrollment, patient and professional educational information, program registration, patient satisfaction surveys, and appointment scheduling and reminders can be added. Clinical applications could include prescription refill services, drug interaction information and treatment protocol reminders. As most of these services can be automated through voice mail or IVR, there is limited impact on the agent/nurse's time; however, personnel should still be available in case patients have additional questions.

Any of these concepts can have integrated network links to the facility's emergency room or to 911 emergency services. A common feature of these current categories, and the most expensive factor, is that nearly all of the calls handled are inbound only. Figure 7.2 illustrates the current, one-way, environment.

Technology and Applications

The most common call center components are automatic call distributors (ACD), IVR units, computer telephony integration (CTI) servers, and video and predictive dialers. While the appropriateness of each technology to each patient segment is not necessarily a given, there are some obvious applications

Figure 7.2. Current Patient Access to Information

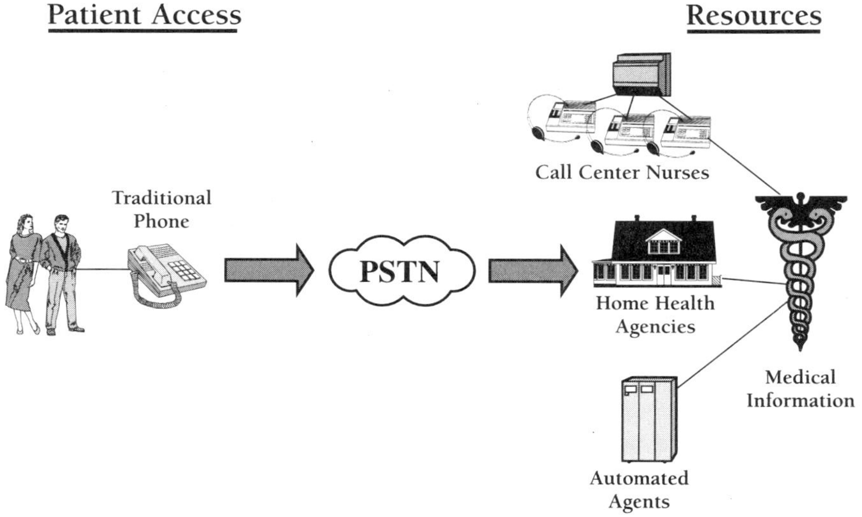

that work best with different technologies. We will look at some common applications that correspond with these technologies as they are deployed and integrated in an MCC. Due to the high level of interest in the Internet, we will also discuss integrating the World Wide Web. Security, reliability, and integration will complete the discussion.

Automatic Call Distributor. The ACD intelligently routes calls based on programmed instructions (e.g., to a welcome recording or an IVR application) until an agent, nurse, or caregiver is available. Today, more sophisticated capabilities can be built in for intelligent or skills-based routing by language, medical specialty, or assigned caregiver. The benefits include:

- Increased call center efficiency and reduced operating costs
- Effective distribution of calls among agents/nurses/caregivers
- Reduced call abandonment rates because patients are kept on the phone with message announcements, voice mail, and IVR
- Real-time monitoring and reports generated on agent/nurse and call activity to improve call center management

Interactive Voice Response. IVR allows the patient to choose routing options, such as entering identifying information for call routing, scheduling an appointment, completing a patient satisfaction survey, or obtaining education materials by interacting with the host database through telephone keypad entries or spoken word. Newer IVR systems allow the administrator to develop graphical user interface (GUI) screen applications through point-and-click facilities. Outbound dialing is also being integrated to the IVR platform. The benefits include:

- Increased call center efficiency and reduced operating costs
- More calls handled with fewer agents/nurses because patients can access information directly
- Lowered call abandon rates, queue times, and call lengths
- Concentration of agents/nurses on complex tasks instead of provision of routine information
- Improved patient satisfaction because the caller has access to such information as insurance coverage, disease state, or an electronic directory of departments and staff

Computer Telephony Integration. CTI uses patient-identifying information to retrieve patient records from the host system database and displays it in a screen pop to the agent/nurse's computer when the call is connected. An additional CTI application is network screen transfer (patient records follow the call as it is transferred from the call center nurse to the appropriate care provider). IVR integration, screen-based telephony, and predictive dialing are also made possible through the CTI server. Benefits include:

- Increased call center efficiency and reduced operating costs
- Information retrieval by patients without the assistance of an agent/nurse
- Improved quality of patient contact; patients perceive that they are known and valued

Predictive Dialers. A predictive dialer allows the call center to program outbound calls to the patient via their medium of choice, i.e., telephone or pager, to provide recorded appointment or medication reminders or to deliver disease management protocols. The predictive dialer can be programmed to automatically adjust its sequence of outbound calls based on agent/nurse availability (having an agent/nurse available could be important if the patient has questions or if real-time disease management program communications are desired). Benefits include:

- Preprogrammed outbound calls, which save agent/nurse time
- Calls delivered based on agent/nurse availability
- Various messages or healthcare applications can be delivered
- Programmed ability to screen out "no" answers, network messages, or answering machines to ensure delivery to the patient

Video/Telemedicine. Telemedicine for homebound patients can be integrated into an MCC. While video images over "plain old telephone service" are delivered via analog lines with low-frame-per-second results, higher bandwidths (e.g., 56 Kbps, integrated services delivery network [ISDN] or asymmetrical digital subscriber line [ADSL]) are becoming available. ADSL will bring almost unlimited bandwidth to the home, simultaneously carrying voice, video, data, and image. Plain old telephone service speeds, however, are often acceptable as long as a friendly, familiar voice is on the other end.

Color video is a valuable tool for the clinician or home nurse in checking the patient's overall condition. Also, the wound healing process can be monitored via video during bandage changes. This could, after training, even be implemented by the patient. High-speed bandwidth is not required to have color, nor is it required for most patients at home. Keep in mind that monitoring, not diagnosis, is the focus of home care; however, early detection of disease is enhanced. Anecdotal studies have indicated that elderly patients often look forward to the "visit" over video even to the degree that they will do some personal primping before the call. The benefits include:

- Face-to-face contact
- Scalability by size (desktop or room), function, bandwidth, or resolution.
- Reimbursable
- Equipment allowing expert consultation if needed in many large/regional centers

Telemetry Integration. Peripheral medical equipment (e.g., blood pressure cuffs, otoscopes, spirometers, etc.) can be attached to a video or data feed. If the transmission is digital (versus analog) and the receiving equipment in the patient's home has an RS232 port, readings can be sent to the call center which can then be added to the patient record. Benefits include:

- Availability of multiple devices to tailor each patient's monitoring needs
- Immediate display of data on the caregiver's screen and addition to the patient record
- Transmission over telephone lines (i.e., Holter monitors)

Internet/World Wide Web Integration. Internet capabilities allow patients to communicate securely with the caregiver over the Internet. Further integration with other technologies is possible to create multitiered communications using paging, fax, voice mail, or e-mail. There are currently two approaches a Web-enabled call center can use to connect with a patient over the Internet.

1. Web callback (store-and-forward), which involves the patient pressing a button on the Web site, alerting the call center that a callback is requested. Patient information and time to return the call may be included to prepare the calling agent.
2. Web call-through (real-time) which prompts an immediate callback; or depending on the patient's Internet access method and equipment (personal computer, high-speed modem, sound card, microphone, and headset), and assuming a single line connection, Internet voice over data could be used through an Internet telephony gateway infrastructure.

Several organizations have created Web sites for patients to enter personal data and receive selected health information (United Healthcare Optum Health Forums; Blue Cross Blue Shield Anthem). Other sites provide health insurance coverage information or pages for patients to update demographic information or select a new PCP.

As personal Web sites evolve, the call center agent/nurse could deliver disease management protocols or selected information off the Internet directly to the patient's site using push technology. By adding Internet security (e.g., digital envelope) around the patient site, it is made virtually impenetrable.

While most people think of a personal computer as the primary interface to the Internet, screen-based telephones and Web television could become prevalent access tools. Personal Web sites of patients are the norm in this type of environment. Through their Web sites, patients will be able to update demographic information, file insurance claims, change their PCP, or register for educational classes. The caregiver will be able to push the patient's treatment protocols and reminders to the site, download customized education material and pull information off the Internet for delivery. Such technology should be most effective with the chronically ill patient who "walks around" (such as a patient with diabetes) compared with the homebound individual who may prefer direct contact with a caregiver via video.

Security and Reliability. Security issues must be addressed both internally and externally. First, you must protect the integrity of any database information made accessible. Protection of password and personal identification number and determination of organizational policy on the appropriateness of automated delivery of certain information (e.g., cancer test results, HIV test results, etc.) will have to be considered. Second, if your organization decides to employ predictive dialers, you may want to screen your patients regarding family member sensitivities.

Reliability is an issue of vendor selection. How long have they been in business; what is their healthcare embedded base? What is the level of their healthcare knowledge and understanding? What value do you receive from a full-service provider of call center solutions compared with a piecemeal approach to purchase and installation? Other considerations such as open architecture vs proprietary systems, your legacy systems, and your network will affect the overall reliability of any new systems installed.

Computer-Based Patient Record Integration. Managing the patient across the continuum of care is much easier using an MCC approach, provided that there is a data repository for encounters both at the MCC and also in the hospital, physician office, outpatient clinics, and home health agencies. The call center care provider thus has a historical view including the patient's physician and eligibility information as well as the ongoing record.

Patients will have access to this information as well, so that they will know immediately if their request or visit is insured. Satisfaction is increased and claims adjudication decreased because the approval process occurs up front. Billing, appointment scheduling, pharmacy/insurance approval, and medical library access are just some of the applications widely available.

As Figure 7.3 indicates, integrated MCCs of the future will require a "legacy access" database as the source of patient/provider activity. It is created by initially linking the disparate host systems in which relevant patient and administrative information is found and then streaming it into a single repository. Ideally, this will be a database developed specifically for this purpose with its own design, not the existing master patient index. The legacy access database will serve as a buffer to the raw legacy systems and be able to withstand the multiple (often hundreds or thousands) requests it receives each day.

Using medical algorithm software, the patient could be sent to the emergency department immediately, given self-care information, or scheduled for an appointment with the appropriate provider. If the patient is sent to the emergency department, a record of the patient's call can be immediately sent to the hospital to expedite care (be aware that the emergency room personnel may be required by law to obtain the same data in person from the patient).

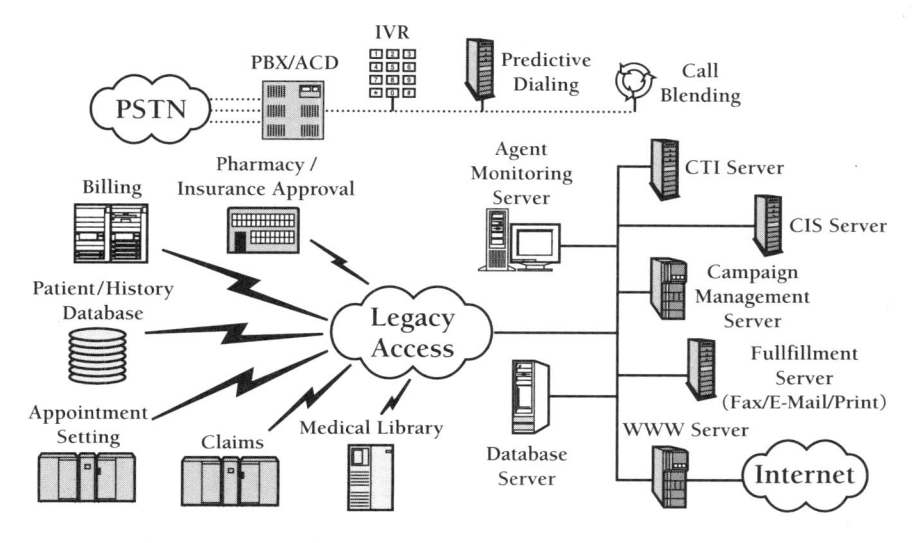

Creating a Vision for Your Medical Call Center 81

Figure 7.3. Medical Call Center of the Future

Source: Versatility Inc., 1998. Used by permission.

If a physician's visit is necessary, the patient will be given appointment information and the medical record can be transferred directly to the physician's office.

Health risk assessments can easily be administered through an MCC. It will be critical to ask questions of the patient to determine a benchline for care and progress. Often this can be done interactively at various intervals. If the Internet is used as a communication mechanism with the patient, questions can be posted on the patient's Web site. Questionnaires can be administered at once or spread out over time. Either way, the provider creates a patient profile against which progress and specific disease management programs are measured. This is the first step to patient stratification which is eminent if you are going to implement disease and/or personal health management plans. This stratification will also provide you with the template for designing and deploying the electronic needs of your center and the patient's home. This could include video, Internet, or medical telemetry equipment.

Disease management programs can be administered through the MCC at various levels depending on patient type and illness severity. Increasingly, health systems are purchasing or creating their own disease-specific programs for this purpose.

PCPs design care protocols for their patients which rely on the patient's willingness and ability to comply. Unfortunately, extremely high noncompliance rates (often up to 60 percent) with medication are the norm. By forming partnerships with the PCP, healthcare systems can identify the proper care protocols for their patients, automate them in the MCC, and measure outcomes effectively across patient populations.

Treatment compliance can be managed using different methods that depend on the sophistication of the communication technology being used. Using a video link to the patient's home, "on-air" appointments can be scheduled to coincide with the frequency with which the patient is to take medication. Wrist devices that alert patients to repeat the medicine dosage can be linked to the system. If the system is interactive, patients can notify the MCC when ready for medication.

An example of motivational patient monitoring is to issue a pharmacy member card to the patient. Every time medicine is refilled, a period of free long-distance telephone service is provided via a rechargeable prepaid card.

Home monitoring can vary according to illness severity and need for occasional or 24–hour observation. In the former, it is common to preschedule appointments and only "visit" at those times. In a 24–hour situation, video may be the answer. In either case, the communication is interactive so that patients can initiate calls.

Personal health management programs are usually developed from health risk assessment instruments, patient feedback, illness severity analysis, and PCP care protocols. Combining this information with behavioral research and appropriate MCC technology can be a powerful way to create an effective behavior/medicine modification program.

Charting goals—nutritional, exercise regimen, or psychological—with the patient is critical for measuring progress and providing counseling if goals are not met.

Providing the patient with disease-specific information is also an essential component of any successful program. Multiple information delivery avenues can be used including educational radio, books on tape, research articles, daily health updates, self testing, videos, and disease management review.

When implementing these new technologies with the wide variations of applications already in place, attention to your integration strategy is vital. You want users to have these features all linked to your legacy systems. Choosing an integration partner will be one of your most important decisions. Consider the following tasks when selecting that partner.

- Assessing needs
- Creating the application scope
- Identifying resources and responsibilities
- Developing roles and responsibilities
- Gathering initial functional specifications
- Developing technical specifications
- Developing preliminary product solution
- Creating an end-to-end project plan
- Managing projects

Creating a Vision for Your Medical Call Center 83

- Performing technical integration of components
- Developing application interface or review of the third-party development
- Developing turnover procedure
- Developing and implementing training plans
- Providing timetables and milestone charts

Additional features like audiotext, text-to-speech, simultaneous voice-over-data, and enhanced fax will simplify the delivery of information and maximize use of the network.

Outsourced or In-House

Once your organization has made the decision to provide patient services through a call center, your next question is: "Do we build an in-house department or outsource the service?" It is projected that by 2000, most mid-size (200–500 beds) and large (500+ beds) hospitals and healthcare integrated delivery systems, managed care organizations and payers will own, operate, or outsource MCC services. Some of these organizations could conceivably provide the services themselves to smaller hospitals and medical practices.

Current trends show a 50/50 split between those building in-house capabilities and those outsourcing. The trend should shift slightly toward outsourcing during the next two to three years, but by 2000 shift back to in-house services as technology costs and in-house expertise grow. The pros and cons of in-house versus outsourcing are listed in Table 7.1.

Selling the Vision

MCC technology and applications are limitless, and the opportunities are plentiful. The challenge is selling the concept of these opportunities to top management, who alone can allocate the resources to transform the vision into operational reality.

To sell the vision, you must demonstrate that the MCC adds value to your organization and its partners. Often, "added value" translates into both customer service improvements and cost savings. In the absence of specific contractual arrangements with managed care plans, the nurse triage and wellness call centers must substantiate predicted cost savings by collecting "prior inclination" data from callers. That is, callers must be asked what they would have done had the call center nurse not been available to them. An average savings based on the difference between the intended action and original inclination must be calculated. Although these data are often perceived as "soft," they are invaluable in discussions about savings.

Medical guidelines and computer-based protocols provide the following clear and rapid clinical benefits for a nurse triage call center.

Table 7.1. Comparison of In-House and Outsourced Call Center Service

In-House	Outsourced
Pros	Pros
Can offer more personalized service	Eliminates capital expenditure
Greater control over service quality	Flexible pricing (per call, flat fee. pmpm)
Ability to customize services to local market needs	Experience
Can generate service bureau revenues	Can launch multiple services simultaneously
Can generate outbound health plan delivery revenue	
Lower cost over time	
Cons	Cons
Initial capital expenditure	Up front set up costs
7 x 24 staffing requirements	More expensive over time
Training of staff / learning curve of staff	Potentially limited functionality (i.e. inbound only)
Phase in individual service separately	Lack local knowledge
Account department / management requirements	Lack of data integration
	Standardized procedures and protocols

- Appropriate utilization of healthcare resources
- Standardized documentation
- Consistent advice
- Increased patient/physician satisfaction
- Reduced liability
- Fewer unnecessary visits to the emergency department

A wellness call center reinforces your commitment to building strong working relationships with health partners and provides information that helps the population at large in making wise healthcare decisions. It offers an opportunity to build relationships with major managed care partners in demand/utilization management as well as in managing the health (rather than disease) of member populations. Individual callers and the population at large can count on the wellness call center for up-to-date and accurate information about health, making it a valuable resource for the community.

Securing buy-in data for an administrative call center requires documentation to demonstrate cost savings, an acceptable pay-back period, improved customer service, and service levels. Most of the cost savings are generated from centralization which improves productivity and consequent full-time equivalent savings. It is important to present an organized and accurate plan for centralization. Documentation must demonstrate an acceptable pay-back period; demonstrate how the center will improve service levels and customer service by improving average speed of answer and reducing both call processing times and abandonment rates; and show support from the departments that will manage the call center.

Before going to executive management with a plan, get buy-in data from internal information services and telecommunications departments. The executive team's financial support may turn the dream into reality, but it will take the long-term support of your organization's technical departments to keep the dream alive.

Summary

MCC technologies and applications that can have a positive impact on managed care delivery are almost limitless. As you determine your vision, be sure to have in mind the following questions: (1) Do you simply want an efficient front end for receiving calls? (2) Do you want to offer triage services? (3) Is your organization ready for a fully functional "electronic physician's office?"

Understand your organization's strategy. Where are you going, not only today but five years from now? That information is essential to determine your vision. Once established, your vision will help determine what you need and whether you should build or outsource. Vendors will assist in cost/benefit analysis of their equipment, but do not lose sight of internal factors such as "prior inclination" costs in the case of a nurse triage program. The technology is available to take your vision to its outer reaches. With the projected increase in utilization of call center services, don't let your organization be left behind!

About the Authors

Julie L. Barr is System Director for the Samaritan Call Center, Samaritan Health System, Phoenix, Arizona.

Sue Laufenberg is Director of Marketing, Sprint Healthcare Systems Inc., Overland Park, Kansas.

Brian L. Sieckman is Demand Management Marketing Manager, Sprint Healthcare Systems Inc.

Developing Web-Based Knowledge Management Systems for Healthcare Call Centers

John R. Odden

Introduction

This article describes my experience with a long-time client who implemented a proprietary business application that was designed for and employed in a centralized call center. The application included several leading edge technologies along with some complex business logic for very advanced transaction processing. When the call center opened, the new agents, extensively trained in telephone transactions, had to struggle to respond to nontransaction inquiries. Instead of using ring binders containing policies and procedures, the more successful agents referred to sticky notes on their computer monitors, little stacks of three-by-five cards on their desks, or crib sheets pinned to the walls of their workspaces. The less successful agents did not have these aids, but sometimes borrowed them from their coworkers.

Project leaders in the new telephone service center provided the project with its objective: "To deliver a knowledge management tool that would work around the transaction system and provide ready access to the information in the ring binders." My client had scheduled enhancements well into the future, and was determined to impose no risk on the transaction system and to meet the established timeline for improvements.

The project team decided to use Web technology on the corporate intranet to deploy the knowledge management tool. Other choices may have led to the achievement of our objective, but they would not have commanded the same level of enthusiasm. Even today one wonders whether using Web technology ensured the success of the project, simply because it is the "hot thing" and so many information technology professionals consider themselves established or aspiring "Internet experts."

The project included call center teams that felt they had neither the time nor the resources needed to build more sophisticated knowledge bases. The Web-enabled approach first arose as a straw model to dig out the pros and cons of a more formal, rigorous approach. Call center agents and their leaders responded to the use of Web technology with enthusiasm and supported the creation and incremental improvement of prototype knowledge base content.

Knowledge Management

Although knowledge management has its roots in knowledge engineering work with case-based reasoning and neural networks, the project team adopted the definition used by the telephone service representatives, supervisors, and managers in the call center. For them, the reference documents used to conduct transactions and answer questions constitute their "knowledge library." They formed a team to consider options for migrating the knowledge library from a traditional paper-based approach to some form of a computer-based system.

The team considered multiple alternatives including packaged software products. To be successful, their "knowledge management system" had to accommodate text-based content authored and maintained using desktop word processing or publishing applications. Indeed, these traditional sources of knowledge continue to be published, distributed, and updated via paper to serve an extensive user community outside the call center. This practice is expected to continue for a long time.

The fact that this knowledge library is principally available as highly formatted text posed a significant problem for the project. The call center was not staffed to take on data conversion as an initial or ongoing task. The team considered the possibility of assigning this responsibility to the subject matter experts (SMEs) who authored the knowledge library material. However, the SMEs were spread geographically and organizationally throughout a very large enterprise and included a significant proportion of senior specialists with demanding roles and responsibilities in the business. In fact, SME "buy-in" to any approach to automation of the knowledge library loomed large as an obstacle to change.

To solve this problem, the call center planned to build templates for each major type of knowledge library content. Early content releases depended on focusing on the priority of the information and the practical ability of the responsible SME community to to deliver core content and periodic updates. The decision to use Web tools and Web formats did not make things easy. But it did not hurt either. The fact that team members could rapidly modify the appearance and navigation of the knowledge library helped to create considerable enthusiasm. Mistakes in the format or suggestions for improvement were minor items that could be changed relatively quickly and easily.

Knowledge Workers. Call center agents are knowledge workers who apply skill and expertise to successfully complete telephone transactions. Some, notably advice nurses, are clinically certified. Selection criteria include measurable skill levels; training and testing are rigorous. Agents often apply advanced concepts and vocabulary as they acquire and evaluate information from the caller, available transaction systems, and databases. Knowledge base information may enter into this mix, either in the form of selected policies and procedures, or as guidelines, scripts, practices, or recommendations. The call center agent must rapidly assess the transaction, identify relevant guiding practices, and communicate efficiently and professionally with the caller.

Transactions with limited inputs and predetermined outputs are often directed to interactive voice response or Web sites. This allows call center agents to handle transactions that demand skilled, real-time application of knowledge and knowledge bases. It also reduces the likelihood of errors in gathering the inputs because a live agent can make errors in keying in a response on a very simple transaction.

Subject Matter Experts. In common practice, the interpretations applied to particular transactions, queries, or situations are found in policy or procedure manuals that codify the facts, decision criteria, and actions. The principal contributors to these manuals were SMEs, the internal resources who supported knowledge workers. Call center agents also knew certain SMEs who were formally or informally available to receive and respond to calls when situations arose which required expertise.

With Web-based knowledge management, the goal was to turn the SMEs into electronic publishers, making it very simple to notify knowledge workers of important updates. With updates deposited in password-secured folders in the intranet, the next mouse click requesting a piece of the knowledge base generates the correct, updated content. In an added benefit, SMEs responding to queries from knowledge workers about missing or unclear information or exceptions to stated practice can make changes and corrections immediately. This compressed cycle of interaction between the knowledge workers and the SMEs generates a new relationship, an electronic connection that enables the SMEs to be considerably more responsive to the real needs of the business. There are also no more racks of paper manuals, even for new knowledge workers who are trained in Web-based knowledge resources during orientation.

The Approach

Defining Requirements. For this project, we modified the requirement criteria to take advantage of the capabilities of Web-based tools. Enterprise standards for the browser and server guided the choice of tools for constructing the knowledge base. User interface standards for the call center environment, modified in accordance with typical Internet design practices, established the targeted look and feel. The only decision needed to launch the project was to select a topic or content focus for the pilot. Given the urgency of the situation confronted by the client, a rapid deployment approach was used (Table 8.1).

Resisting the obvious temptation to go for the big win, less complex content was opted for, whereby SMEs were interested in participating in a new

Table 8.1. Nine Steps to a Successful Project

A simple approach that yields quick results while building team skills and confidence can a be good way to start. We've had success with these steps.

1. Work with an initial management sponsor to identify a potential topic for a Web-enabled knowledge base. Balance the feasibility of finding content and motivated team members with the natural desire to score a big win with the first effort.
2. Solicit and/or appoint initial members to the rapid deployment team. Members to be recruited include a project facilitator, a few call center agents, possibly a supervisor, SMEs appropriate to the pilot topic, a proven digital artist, and a Web developer.
3. Convene a meeting to charter the team and get the proposed members on board. Release those who cannot commit to meet regularly to critique and improve the knowledge base, or who are clearly not going to be comfortable with a rapid deployment approach that treats team members as equals.
4. Set the date and time for the initial team work session allowing the digital artist one week to prepare a prototype from the time the SMEs provide the initial batch of sample content.
5. Conduct a review and improvement session on schedule. Start with whatever the digital artist has formatted within the established time frame. Emphasize the view of the agents and supervisors regarding the formats, icons, and priorities for building content that will streamline their ability to render rapid and accurate customer service. Stimulate a discussion about the pros and cons of various formats, color schemes, and navigation icons. Schedule another review cycle for the following week. Prioritize content gathering and formatting efforts with an ear to agent feedback. Good call center agents know where the gaps are in their information environment. A useful Web-enabled knowledge base will fill those gaps rather than repeating material that is already available in other systems.
6. Before the last review cycle, bring in a user interface expert with training and experience in a formal approach to assessing ease of use and quality of design. Fold feedback from the user interface assessment into creation of the final templates for the last review meeting.
7. Recruit a member of the rapid deployment team or a successful agent or supervisor to lead an agent training program. Make the project facilitator, digital artist, and Web developer available to the trainer to build a brief overview of the knowledge base and its use.
8. Have the developer set up the knowledge base in a preproduction environment and simulate hits approximating the peak workload of the call center, plus a safety factor. Run such a stress test during a weekend or off-shift period or over a few days in an isolated environment. Set up a few workstations in the production environment with access to the preproduction Web server. Have the agent members of the rapid cycle team serve as beta test users of the pilot knowledge base content. While Web technology tends to be robust and scalable, it is always best to test everything.
9. Provide a help desk for the day you plan to go live. Not everyone is comfortable with the Web surfing style of user interface; and not every desktop software roll-out is perfect. Provide reasonable support at the start to reduce stress for everyone involved. Wait a while to see what works and what does not in the pilot. Then form a team to define and work on the next phase of your Web-enabled knowledge base.

approach to knowledge management. The project team decided to focus on a successful team experience highlighting the simplicity and speed of the Web-based approach. We were convinced that using intranet tools for knowledge management is different from "building a Web site" and different from deploying a sophisticated knowledge engineering system.

For the pilot, it was planned to assemble the team in two weeks. It was determined whether the managers were prepared to spend the time needed to enlist appropriate and motivated team members. Some professionals who initially volunteered to work with "that cool Web technology" were found to be not too eager to join in, after a candid discussion of roles, responsibilities, and the process. Finding the right group takes time.

In fairness to the team, it was pointed out that the rapid deployment method and/or the Web-enabled technology might not be effective. The purpose of the pilot was to demonstrate whether and how well this approach worked for their particular business area and knowledge base. It was stressed that quickly finding out that more traditional knowledge engineering tools were required or that there was no source to build a knowledge base would be as valid and valuable a result as creating a powerful new tool. In my judgment, setting realistic expectations and responding in a flexible way to any issues that arose helped the team gain confidence.

Once the method was determined to be effective, the next objective was to learn how to function as a team in building a knowledge base that would enhance the productivity of the call center agents. A manager who intends to build a large knowledge base by sponsoring a number of teams or phases of rapid deployment work would do well to consider the potential role of unique style or even whimsy in creating the eventual knowledge base. There are many reasons why a Web-enabled knowledge base is more effective than several ring binders full of valuable content. To some extent, voluminous paper references are handicapped by the quality of the index and table of contents. Navigation to the right information in a set of ring binders is not guaranteed. The same fact applies to a Web-enabled knowledge base. However, it is fairly simple to use icons, color, and even animation when formatting Web-enabled content. A team that is given the freedom to experiment and innovate with the design and navigation options of Web content is more likely to build an effective knowledge base.

Prototyping and Iterating. Given the client's need to have a knowledge management tool in place quickly, a rapid, user-focused method was used to build energetic teams and fast-track the results. Simply put, the knowledge base content and formatting options were reviewed and discussed, prototypes of the options were created, the prototypes were critiqued, and then the cycle was repeated. With a facilitator who understood the functional business area and the transactions that are served in the call center, the team included SMEs who were the process and content experts responsible for authoring the electronically published knowledge base; skilled agents involved in the content, format, and navigation that would optimize their access to the knowledge base; a digital artist who provided tailored icons and alternative content formats; and developers who assisted in configuring the browser and Web server to deliver the content consistently and rapidly.

Although four or five iterations of the cycle are generally adequate, we were prepared in this project to complete seven or more iterations to ensure that content was optimized and that call center agents and supervisors would view it with enthusiasm. Each iteration was conducted over a period ranging from 3 to 10 days, based on the workload in the call center, the effort needed to acquire and format initial content into sample templates or prototypes, and the availability of key team members. The SMEs were busy senior professionals, and we knew that neither they nor the call center members were in a position to abandon all other duties to build a Web-enabled knowledge base.

The Results

Off-the-shelf software programs were used in this project, including Web browsers and a Web server (Table 8.2). The content was prototyped, reviewed, critiqued, and modified until the agents who would look at it time and again for eight or more hours every day declared that it was "right." A digital artist was available during each rapid cycle to revise formats and create special icons. If an alert or a sensitive item called for a special announcement, the digital artist used color or other visuals to provide the needed effect. Some requests seemed a bit unusual, even radical. For example, although it seemed that the standard browser navigation toolbar would be immediately accepted as a clean and efficient interface, the project team accepted the possibility that the call center agents facing the same thing day after day might come up with a different answer, which they certainly did! The navigation icons eventually developed were appealing, but very different.

Several navigation interfaces were suggested and prototyped, with different visual metaphors for access to the knowledge base. Team members who were call center agents clearly preferred a two-dimensional interface, quite different from what team members with formal information technology training and experience expected. On this interface, the most frequently referenced information is represented in a two-dimensional visual format, with an alphabetic index on the vertical coordinate and a "hot features" index on the horizontal coordinate. This interface was adopted, consistent with the project approach.

In this approach, the work was chartered for the benefit of the call center agents, and entries for the knowledge library were gathered and formatted according to the expressed priorities of the agents. The goal was to give the agents something easier and friendlier to work with than three-ring binders, and to spare them the burden of receiving, opening, and inserting the stream of updates to the multiple reference manuals used in their daily job—completing transactions and answering questions over the telephone.

Developing Web-Based Knowledge Management Systems 93

Table 8.2. Web Technologies

Browser
A Web browser enables the desktop personal computer user to use the intranet to access information. Because intranet technologies tend to have vendor-specific features when first released, I recommend using a standard desktop image across the enterprise, or at least through the call center. With a standard image and browser (including a uniform version level), the knowledge base content can take advantage of every desirable formatting and navigation feature. If multiple browsers are in use, the content and navigation will have to fall back to a "least common denominator" of features that work alike on every desktop; the digital artist who builds knowledge base content will face unnecessary challenges.

Web Server
Usually the enterprise standard Web server powering the intranet can support knowledge management in the call center. Detailed engineering and telecommunication/computer protocols may be required to support computer telephony integration and special features like "screen pops" that speed up call handle time. Even with an automated knowledge base, it takes time to get to the content to handle a specific call. With the caller's patient identifier or transaction type entered into a voice response unit before the call is transferred, the Web server can "push" appropriate knowledge base content to pop up on the agent's screen.

Data Formats
A foundation element for the internet, hypertext markup language (HTML) is the scripting language that controls the format of information displayed in a Web browser window. Because call centers usually have very little knowledge base content in HTML format at the start of a project, one of their first choices must be to convert content into HTML or to use a "plug-in" or other browser feature that can convert the format to HTML on the fly. Current experience shows that large pieces of content convert slowly. If real-time performance is a key objective, it is better to convert formats to HTML at the time of publication rather than with every access to the knowledge base.

When the first phase of content was completed, reviewed, and tested, the pilot roll-out commenced with the normal anxiety that accompanies such an event. The training needed was less than that anticipated, and team members volunteered to assist with training during the roll-out. Early feedback was positive. The core transaction processing application continued to run successfully without any interference from the knowledge management tool. Call center agents were able to find and use the information. Approximately two months of intense effort created a successful initial installment of the call center knowledge library. Successive phases of activity, each equally brief, yielded a complete knowledge base.

Lessons Learned

Transferring external paper-based knowledge resources to desktop computers via the intranet can simplify the work load of call center agents. Agents can access needed information by pointing and clicking instead of leafing through ring binders. Web-enabled technology can eliminate the need to change the knowledge base access points and content for healthcare applications. This is no small gain, given the complexity of modifying applications that often have embedded knowledge bases, knowledge engineering algorithms, and demanding requirements for interfaces and integrity.

Even when searching is restricted to a short list of critical keywords, a Web-based knowledge management application is more efficient for call center agents. The efficiencies realized depend on the particular transaction mix handled by the agents and how frequently they access the knowledge base to obtain information needed to complete a transaction or respond to a customer inquiry. Although business owners of healthcare call centers are quick to appreciate shorter times to handle calls, they typically are reluctant to publicize performance impact measures. This reflects the perception on their part that an effective call center constitutes a meaningful business advantage.

Starting with a pilot phase and setting realistic goals help the project team gain confidence and gauge their ability to define and build content. The experience of the pilot phase sets the stage for productive discussions among call center leaders regarding the value of building new content templates and acquiring updated, effectively formatted content to add to the knowledge base.

Putting a few strong call center agents on the project team helps capture the perspective of what knowledge management means on the frontline of customer service. Effective call center agents develop a body of knowledge and are very confident about what they need to do their job efficiently. The templates, formatting, and navigation tools created based on agent input are not necessarily what the project manager or SMEs expect.

The Future

As always, the future will take its time in coming, and some organizations will continue pre-Web practices. Even if a knowledge library is not automated, call center agents do have tools, including three-ring binders and other resources, like the personal stack of three-by-five cards. Paper will also continue to be a factor, as recognized by my client, for various reasons, including legal and regulatory requirements.

Automated Systems. Other scenarios exist with automated systems. For example, some legacy applications offer online access to policies and procedures or integrate knowledge base access into a business processing system. In essence, these applications supply a complete set of tools for call center agents and other customer service and transaction handling centers. If system maintenance is affordable and business needs are met, there is no need to make changes. Indeed, the ideal scenario for knowledge management is integrated access to the knowledge base from the transaction processing system, accompanied by context-sensitive access to the relevant (or well-chosen, priority-ranked) knowledge detail. There is no reason to not integrate knowledge management into a newly designed, developed, or procured business application other than the additional time and expense required to deliver the expanded functionality. (Use caution, however; these costs may be considerable.)

Some recently designed, multitiered client/server applications include knowledge management functionality. This can be fully integrated or provided by a parallel function working alongside a core transaction processing system. I recommend conducting a cost/benefit analysis to determine whether the benefits associated with knowledge management justify the costs of deploying an advanced tool with knowledge engineering or case-based reasoning capabilities. Knowledge library access can also be woven into a transaction system in the form of scripts that guide agents in what to say to callers at each step of a particular transaction. Although script pushing systems may not seem sophisticated, the branching and options in a script-driven system may indeed reflect an effective, complete implementation of knowledge management.

Finally, there are now desktop tools that can support knowledge management requirements. Although such a solution can be configured to work in a call center environment, it cannot by definition be scaled to support multiple call center agents working in one or more service centers. Web-based approaches are of interest because they can be prototyped and developed on desktop systems and subsequently migrated to appropriate servers to achieve performance, reliability, and other operational criteria.

These capabilities and, indeed, this experience have convinced me that Web-enabled knowledge management will have a strong future. Vendors continue to offer new Web software components and "Web interfaces." Call centers clearly can benefit from such tools which prevent call center agents leafing through bound paper references while they struggle to respond to queues of callers waiting for service.

There are also other tools, methods, and algorithms for knowledge management which can add speed, accuracy, and effectiveness to the kind of Web-enabled knowledge base described in this article. We are eagerly watching the marketplace and assessing new advances in Web-compatible tools that may offer new opportunities to deliver the full value of the emerging intranet computing paradigm.

About the Author

John R. Odden is a director for First Consulting Group, where he is a member of Network Integration Services.

Developing A Successful Call Center: One Hospital's Story

Donna M. Campbell

Sarasota Memorial Hospital (SMH) is a 70-year-old acute-care facility located on Florida's west coast. The third largest public hospital in the state, with 853 beds, SMH implemented its medical call center in August 1994. The call center strategy uses the most efficient systems possible and complements the hospital's goal of becoming one of the nation's top 25 hospitals by the year 2000. The center initially blended an existing physician referral program and private branch exchange (PBX) services with new "telenurse" triage. Within a short time centralized community class registration and recorded health information lines were added. The resulting call center was branded The Health Resource Network (THRN).

Why Create a Call Center?

Our research verified that there are numerous reasons to start a call center. Convincing management of its advantages is not as difficult as it once was. After all, the concept of a demand management call center is not new. The term "demand management" has even been trademarked.

In the case of SMH, merging call functions that were previously handled by the telecommunications and marketing departments provided economies of scale. Nurse call services and recorded messages extended a community service that generates goodwill and expands patient education programs. Using local neighborhoods or any other parameter set, system reports track a caller's response to hospital marketing efforts. The call center can be proven to generate revenue. When THRN is the first point of patient contact with our facility, and an admission results, that revenue is considered to be THRN-generated. (Actual revenue received is credited, naturally, to the service providing departments.) Another purpose of establishing our call center was, and continues to be, cost avoidance. Medical problems that undergo triages via telephone result in fewer unnecessary visits to our emergency care and minor care centers. This reduces the hospital's costs and saves the patient time and expense. Processing of appropriate patients is then accelerated in those emergency centers.

Expanding Successful Programs

With those benefits in mind, SMH established a call center mission "to delight the caller." This would be accomplished "by building stronger relationships through comprehensive telephone-based health information and physician referral services."

Development of an operational plan required the cooperation of the telecommunications, planning, and marketing departments. This included:

- A pro forma, and operational and capital budgets
- Selection of medical protocol and scheduling software vendor
- Coordination of selected software with hardware and telecommunications systems
- Formation of a physician advisory committee to review written triage protocols
- Organizational structure and reporting responsibilities
- Job descriptions and pay grades
- Telephone competencies
- Formal guidelines and procedures
- Existing staff orientation and training on the software
- Recruitment and training of new staff
- Space allocation and renovations
- Obtaining furniture, supplies, and equipment

Next we embarked on a major space expansion and renovation project that would consolidate several work locations into a single call center. The staff was included in blueprint review and color scheme selection. Enhancements such as adjustable keyboards, personal computer monitor hoods, foot rests, and personal lighting were selected. A special textured wallpaper was chosen to improve acoustics, as were paneled workstations. The call center also includes ample space for storing reference materials; a well-lighted work room with fax, copy machine, and place for collating materials; and a modern break room. The hospital's "Command Center" is situated in the call center. Designed to accommodate senior management during a disaster situation, the spacious room provides multiple telephone and personal computer access, three televisions, video teleconferencing capabilities, multiple white boards, and storage.

From its beginning nearly four years ago, the main campus call center was designed to provide a "one call does it all" service to our county's population of more than 300,000 citizens. PBX operators were cross-trained on "Centra-Max," a National Health Enhancements System software. This gave nonclinician telephone service representatives (TSRs) and PBX operators the ability to provide service referrals and registration information. The center's functional organization chart provided for the addition of physician's appointment scheduling and outbound "After Care" nurse call functions as the call center grew.

Developing A Successful Call Center 99

Although a number of minor issues confronted the call center from its inception, one major challenge faced THRN—obtaining necessary advertising to increase calls, thereby justifying additional staff. Management understandably did not want to vigorously market THRN's services until staffing levels were capable of handling resulting calls. Yet, without aggressive marketing, call volume initially remained low. It did not support the addition of TSRs. This challenge was gradually resolved as hospital-wide confidence in the program increased and promotional dollars, though limited, drove call volume upward.

Another consideration in establishing our call center was the initial reluctance of some hospital departments to relinquish their own class scheduling responsibilities and patient follow-up calls. THRN was a new, unproved department. Creating trust was bound to take time. Without a strong commitment from the departments that we attempted to serve, the THRN staff struggled to increase business. Accepting small assignments and building on its successes, the call center eventually overcame the barrier. Most departments are now not only willing but eager to off-load some of their work volume to THRN. Thus both service referrals and class registration volumes have increased.

Staffing and Volume

Initially SMH computed THRN's staffing levels to provide medical call center coverage Monday through Friday, 8 AM until 5 PM. One nurse and two TSRs were capable of handling physician referrals, health information, phone triage, and a portion of class registrations for the start-up function. Later, 13 PBX operators were cross-trained to provide back-up support. The night operator fills her down-time by producing confirmation letters to class enrollees and printed health information. Before THRN even attempted to take patient calls, the program was publicized in-house. Articles in the hospital's newsletter and flyers helped spread the word. Reminders were included in the special message section of pay vouchers, and an Open House showcased the modern new facility. Our staff accepted triage calls and health information requests from SMH's employees for six weeks before our "go-live" date. This permitted us to test systems, correct deficits, redefine training needs, and build speed in working with the software.

Despite our in-house trial, several problems were not discovered until after the center began accepting outside calls. Most significantly, our PBX technology could not suitably accommodate switching from the hospital's mainframe access and CentraMax. The time required to "bring up" the software for class scheduling or service referrals significantly slowed response to other in-bound calls. More technologically advanced products were available by this time, which, however, required a large investment. Like most hospital call centers, we jockey for capital equipment dollars along with direct patient care departments. Our "budget crunch" prevented expensive system redesign. Therefore,

THRN was required to revamp the "one call does it all" program. We assigned employees to either PBX or THRN duties on a rotating basis. Cross-training permits the entire staff to fill in in any area of the call center where needed. It also gives employees current product line knowledge.

Growing

By Fall 1996, SMH increased the telephone triage portion of THRN to a 24-hour-a-day, seven-day-a-week (24 x 7) operation by outsourcing overflow calls. Our outsource agreement required an easily obtainable minimum number of calls to the back-up service every month. There is also a charge per call. The extensive call reports from the overflow service verified that public demand for this service was steadily increasing. Because our population was already familiar with "Ask a Nurse" type programs (and despite the limited professional promotion), call volume continues to build by word of mouth.

THRN has since added another full-time nurse. An additional nonclinician handles registrations and product fulfillment for the hospital's membership program entitled "Passport." A part-time nurse augments daytime outbound calls. A full-time database assistant was hired to update files, physician profiles, and perform service referral input. A system power user dedicated to perform these functions is essential and should be included in the original pro forma of any medical call center.

Statistical reviews indicate that the vast majority of our referrals are for internal medicine and family practice physicians. Predictably, a high percentage of our medical information calls in Florida are regarding skin cancer. This results in a high number of dermatologist referrals. Our recorded health information lines receive a varying number of calls each month. Fluctuation of call volume is caused partly by public response to "hot" topics such as an outbreak of encephalitis or measles. Our most frequently accessed recorded tapes are mental health topics, men's health, and digestive information. Not coincidentally, the problem that requires triage most commonly is stomach disorders. We observe higher usage of the lines, understandably, when an advertising campaign promotes the service to the community. Although Florida experiences short, mild winters, the advent of the flu season brings additional calls to both the recorded health line and the nurse triage service. Since Sarasota also welcomes a large tourist influx in the winter, a transitory population uses our various telephone medical information services. Often these "winter visitors" need local physicians and healthcare advice because their personal physicians are located in their home states.

Quantity Standards

THRN set standards for call waiting, talk times, wrap times, and call abandoned rates based both on the staff's growing understanding of our local caller demographics and on nationwide call center benchmarking. Factors such as seasonal business and community health interests must be considered when realistic performance targets are set and adjusted periodically. Staff participation in target setting should be encouraged. Employees are more likely to strive to meet goals they help to set. (Our staff still reviews the 3 percent abandon rate target to determine if THRN should "raise the bar" on expectations.) Initially our target was an average talk time of four minutes. However, the average age of our population in Southwest Florida requires our staff to work with an older population. This results in longer-than-average talk times when our representatives provide reassurance and confirmation of information to them. Our average talk time runs about six minutes, excluding wrap-up time. We have dedicated ourselves to the goal of complete caller satisfaction; we do not rush calls through in favor of higher productivity. Still, THRN manages to maintain an abandoned call rate of well under 10 percent; however, I know of other centers that accept a 20 percent or higher abandoned call rate. The acceptable call loss target varies nationally. Once again, the establishment of appropriate targets for level of service must be based on sound knowledge of the population served.

Biweekly reports are made using a comprehensive management tool which measures and times overall call center activities. Productivity and cost per unit of service are tracked. Monitoring call reports helps THRN to predict call volumes for tourist seasons and upcoming call campaigns as well as monitor overall call center costs. It is easy to become carried away with statistics. One caveat: manage the data; do not let it manage you. One entire full-time equivalent (FTE) employee could easily be used as a department statistician, even in a small call center such as ours. Overcome the urge to create massive reports and charts. The objective should be to find several key measurement factors and track them. Reports should not baffle readers with a plethora of meaningless numbers.

Our inbound calls, including PBX, exceed 100,000 per month, and TSRs provide approximately 1000 registrations every month. SMH has employees, not volunteers, who handle patient condition information. A staff of three FTEs answers 20,000 to 25,000 calls every month. The center receives the most calls on Monday, with Friday being traditionally the slowest day. Peak call hours are between 10 AM and noon and again between 2 PM and 4 PM. The majority of our callers, by a ratio of 2:1, are women. This is predictable because women make the majority of healthcare decisions for their spouses and families.

Quality Standards

THRN developed two surveys to measure the quality of our services: one measures caller satisfaction with our physician referral service and the other documents patient education and tracks satisfaction with the nurse triage component. Surveys sent to callers are postage-paid, preaddressed to the

THRN director. The nursing staff has also worked closely with a physician advisory committee to develop additional medical protocols that augment the already extensive software package. These physicians conduct annual reviews of all protocols and review irregular triage calls or reported problems. In addition, staff members meet regularly to conduct case studies of actual calls. This ensures that medical protocols are followed at all times. The committee steered organizational activities for THRN for its first two years. Once the protocols were approved, the physician advisory committee dissolved. Today we refer physician-related complaints to the hospital's medical affairs office.

Time to Fine-Tune

After our second year of operation we reevaluated the quality and service indicators that had served us well since inception. Shift management reports showed predictable patterns of call volumes that strengthened forecasting staff needs. We determined that cross-training and improved productivity had eliminated the need for three approved, but unfilled, FTEs. The call center now provides numerous value-added services such as procedure rate information and obstetrics preadmitting calls. These functions increased the number of service units provided by us without adding staff.

Installation of new equipment decreased the time required to process incoming PBX calls. Information updates entered by a dedicated database assistant eliminated considerable duplication of effort.

These slight adjustments alone resulted in an annual cost saving of more than $75,000, proving that continued scrutiny of call center operations can provide impressive results.

Expansion to a Regional Call Center

The success of the main campus call center prompted SMH's interest in a cooperative vendor to expand services in a regional setting. Toward that end, in October 1996, representatives from four south Florida healthcare systems formed a task force to examine the efficiencies that a regional call center could provide. Initially the group established an aggressive time frame of three to four months to bring the concept to reality. Because each representative had other job duties that were primary, the task force could not move ahead without dedicated staff driving the processes. This led to the selection of a project manager, who was completely responsible for developing job descriptions, locating physical space, and preparing a pro forma.

The following year SMH opened a regional call center in a shopping mall two miles from the hospital's main campus. The center presently processes incoming referral, registration, and phone triage functions for Sarasota Memorial and Lee Memorial Hospital in Ft. Myers, Florida. (The other two healthcare systems in the original task force have not yet joined the regional call center.) Consolidating physician referral programs in both hospitals as well as class scheduling in one location provides efficiencies that make the program appealing to both partners. Two THRN nurses and one nonclinician accepted lateral transfers to the regional call center when it opened on October 1, 1997. A director, secretary, database administrator, and additional telephone nurses now complete our regional operational team. The full complement of nurses has eliminated the need for an outsourced overflow service. Physician appointment scheduling services will be added in the future.

The Call Centers Today

Today at SMH's main campus, the remaining registered nurse (RN), plus two new hires, process outbound "After Care" calls to support discharged-patient education and improve patient satisfaction. RNs there also conduct surveys for the emergency care center, diabetes treatment services, and the cardiac program, among others. Their triage skills are necessary to foster patient compliance with discharge instructions. They also answer questions about medications and the healing process that patients might not bring to their care provider's attention if the hospital had not instituted the call. Our nurses access the Internet for medical information. They have used it to contact the World Health Organization on behalf of a caller in another country. After Care supports the Joint Commission on the Accreditation of Healthcare Organizations (JCAHO) focus on discharged patient support and general patient education. Therefore, the hospital has committed to adding more nurses as outbound calls continue to increase.

The main campus call center now provides PBX services, alarm monitoring and response, patient information functions, the Passport membership program, outgoing nurse calls, and a hospital message center. The staff includes a director, supervisor, nurses, operators, a database assistant, and department secretary. Overall volume exceeds 1.3 million calls annually, which includes PBX services. To establish staffing levels required, we use a ratio of one FTE to 10,000 calls annually. This sum is added to the number of staff members needed to provide a baseline 24-hour coverage and account for peak call hours. TSRs are taught to cross-sell hospital services or community workshops to callers who may benefit from them. We consider this to be an extended courtesy to the caller and not a true sales effort. No performance or sales bonuses are offered. Compensation is strictly based on hospital-conducted market analysis. TSRs are paid at the same rate as PBX attendants. Telephone triage nurses are compensated at staff nurse levels, an important factor in recruiting top-notch RNs to the call center. Our regional call center offers the same benefits and compensation package as the main campus call center. We find that the best candidates for TSR positions are flexible people with strong customer service backgrounds. Professionals recruited for telenursing positions should possess excellent communication skills, empathy, and poise; have a varied nursing background; and be computer literate.

We have recently begun applying cultural assessments for our telenurses, based on a model of patient-focused care researched by the Picker/Commonwealth Program for Patient-Centered Care,[1] a program established in 1987 with support from the Commonwealth Fund of New York. During this process formal assessments are developed for nurses to identify major cultural factors that can be important in working with callers from diverse cultural backgrounds. The process embraces a dialogue between nurse and caller in which each provides important, relevant information to the other.

The assessment consists of three processes. First, the nurse solicits information in the callers' own words about their ethnicity, background, and even their patterns of decision making. The callers' preferred language is determined and speech interpreters are engaged when necessary.

Telenurses should also be encouraged to join hospital nurse committees for professional development such as Standards and Practices and participate in hospital preparation for JCAHO surveys.

Networking with nurses on the units adds to telenurses' credibility as "real nurses." It fosters relationships that aid in building the call center's business. Most hospitals have minimal budgets for telenurse education outside the institution. Even with limited dollars, a lead RN or supervisor should attend technical training on the software selected for the call center's use. Even one seminar every year will provide a valuable forum to address healthcare industry issues. Benchmarking is another advantage of regional or national demand management call center conference attendance. Having attended both healthcare-related call center conferences and those offered to any type of industry, I find that those dedicated to healthcare provide the most appropriate information on specific matters of interest. These include telenursing, physician referral, call reports, staff productivity, compensation and rewards, and recruitment and retraining.

Our turnover and burnout rates remain lower than the average in large call centers, which does not necessarily mean that morale is optimal. Morale is continually affected by stress level, compensation, and training. Because of our size, neither the hospital's main call center nor the regional call center employs dedicated trainers. THRN uses a "training partner" approach, starting with TSRs listening in on the phones for several days until a comfort level is achieved. The regional call center provided formal training to the staff before its start date.

Summary

As our call centers continue to respond to changes in the healthcare industry and to customer demand, we understand that it is constantly necessary to reinvent ourselves. The call center industry, is, after all, only about 20 years old. It is constantly responding to technological advances. Medical call center managers must also respond to changes in healthcare delivery. We must keep a vigilant eye on industry trends. While we welcome information on other call centers to help us reformulate our targets, we must always customize information to our local market.

Reference

1. Gerteis M, Edgman-Levitan S, Daley J, et al., ed. *Through the Patient's Eyes: Understanding and Promoting Patient-Centered Care.* San Francisco, Calif: Jossey-Bass; 1987.

About the Author

Donna M. Campbell is Director of the Sarasota Memorial Hospital's call center.

One Ringy Dingy: Call Centers of the Nineties

Gerard M. Nussbaum, MS, CPA, CMA, RCDD;
Star P. Ault, MS, MBA

Introduction

In the current healthcare environment, the pressures associated with costs are continuing to increase. Simultaneously, patient service expectations are increasing. Healthcare organizations are also becoming more sensitive to issues such as market share, managing lifetime costs of care, and wellness-directed efforts. The convergence of these trends is motivating healthcare organizations to seek out tools and techniques to help meet these challenges

Some components of the healthcare business have not changed over the years. Many of the business issues still exist. These include the issues of efficiently using clinical time by ensuring that the patients are on time for their appointments and collecting dues owed to the institution after a service has been provided.

Various technologies, tools, and techniques can assist the institution in meeting some of these challenges. A more recent set of technologies involves the call center. A call center combines telephony, computer, and operational procedures to leverage technology and the time of the staff while improving customer service. Call centers usually include a large room in which rows of agents with telephone headsets sit in front of computer workstations fielding incoming calls and making outbound telephone calls. This is the origin of the call center as developed in the banking and airline industry. In most cases, the physical image of the call center still holds.

As institutions implement call center technology, some of the areas in which benefits are seen include the following.

1. Patient management transactions
   - Responding to patient medical advice inquiries
   - Appointment scheduling
   - Medical advice
   - Prescription refills
   - On-call and page operations for clinical access

2. Business support transactions
   - Facilitation of collections activities
   - Insurance claim updates
   - Insurance coverage changes
   - Eligibility information
3. General information
   - Travel directions
   - Hours of operation
   - Visiting hours

To play a role in the process, management must become better informed on the issues, gain an understanding of the technology, and become a knowledgeable participant. The technology that comprises the call center and ways to leverage integration efforts must be balanced with realistic expectations regarding the appropriate use of call centers; no set of tools or technologies is a panacea to the challenges facing healthcare organizations. Mastering these basic concepts will facilitate the implementation and monitoring of the call center and supporting processes.

This article will first look at some of the major components of a call center, then some of the benefits of a call center will be discussed, and finally some of the larger issues associated with setting up a call center will be examined. A bibliography follows, which lists other material that may prove useful in learning more about call centers.

Call centers were developed primarily in the banking, airline, and hotel industries. Each of these industries viewed the caller as a current or potential customer. As healthcare becomes more competitive and as attention is focused not only on acute, intervention-based care, but on managing the health of a covered population, the callers are no longer just patients, but customers. For this reason as well as other directions in healthcare, we will generally refer to callers as customers, not patients.

Overview of Call Center Technology

Various technical building blocks are used in constructing a call center. Some of these components are foundational, while others serve as second-and third-story components which enhance the basic functionality of the call center. However, all the technology in a call center is useless if the people resources are not designed as carefully as the technology. The importance of the call center personnel notwithstanding, we will first look at the technical building blocks before moving on to the personnel component. Table 10.1 summarizes some of the major technical building blocks of the call center.

The Telephone System—The Core. Call centers were originally created to more efficiently manage inbound and outbound telephone calls. Telephone systems still form the core of the call center. Unless the call center is extremely

Table 10.1. Major Technical Building Blocks of a Call Center

Private branch exchange (PBX)

Automatic call distributor (ACD)

Skills-based routing (SBR)

Integrated voice response (IVR)

Computer telephony integration (CTI)

Fax on demand (FOD)

Web integration

---

small (and this is not usually characteristic of call centers created to support healthcare organizations), the central component of the call center is the private branch exchange (PBX), the system that serves to manage and control a company's internal telephones.

Most institutions already have a PBX in place. The existing PBX often becomes the basis for the initial foray into creating a call center if the institution wishes to demonstrate the viability of the concept. Most of the major PBX vendors are actively pursuing the call center market through a combination of internal product extensions to their PBX and third-party products. However, a call center can place an enormous load on a PBX (both in terms of processing cycles as well as number of ports used) so it is often necessary to dedicate a PBX system to support the call center.

Automatic Call Distributor (ACD). To the PBX, one of the first components implemented is often an ACD system. The ACD, in its simplest form, functions like the teller line at the bank. As calls come in, they are directed to the first available agent. If all the agents are busy, the call is held in a queue until an agent becomes available. While the use of ACD technology is not exceedingly sophisticated, in some institutions, the ability to maintain a call on hold until an agent is available can be a major advance, in terms of customer service, over presenting the customer with a busy signal.

The ACD can be made more sophisticated with simple menus created using the extended features of many ACD software systems. The menu allows the caller to select from among several choices. Based on the user's choice, the system then directs the call to one of many queues. Each queue comprises a group of agents who are best suited to handling the call. For example, a caller to Regional Medical Systems may be faced with three choices: (1) make an appointment; (2) renew a prescription; (3) obtain a referral. Based on the caller's selection, he or she is routed to the queue for the agents with the systems and training to fulfill the type of request the caller has made.

An important design consideration when using ACD menus, or any of the more sophisticated customer-interaction technologies, is the ability of the caller to opt out of the system. This is almost universally implemented by allowing the caller to press zero ("0") at any point and be connected directly with a live agent (they may, however, need to wait in a queue before speaking with the next available agent). Even though people have become more tolerant of automated systems, the inability to reach a person can not only infuriate a customer, but may also be life threatening in a medical emergency. (In many institutions, the first part of the initial greeting heard by all callers includes a statement along the following lines: "If this is an emergency, please hang up and dial 911.")

Skills-Based Routing (SBR). In a large call center, individual agents will possess or develop skills and expertise in a given set of areas. Some of this may come through targeted training, while others may have been brought with them to their job.

In addition, customers call in with a specific set of requirements. The degree to which the call center (people and technology) can match the customer's requirements with the skills and capabilities of the agents has a direct impact on the success of the interaction (as we will discuss later, a successful interaction includes meeting the caller's needs in the most time-efficient fashion). To more completely match the caller's requirements with the capabilities of the agents, many call centers implement SBR.

SBR primarily identifies the salient capabilities by which agents are grouped. A resumé is built for each agent based on his or her mastery of each of the identified characteristics. The resumé is then loaded into the system and based on the requirements of the caller, the call is routed to the best qualified agent. *Best* is a slippery concept and will require some hard choices in designing the SBR system. Usually, institutions start off with a few major skills areas and expand them once they have become comfortable with the functioning of the system.

An example may help clarify SBR. In a major metropolitan area, the ability of the call center to handle callers in a language in which they are comfortable may be a major issue. The institution has also trained some of the agents in the process of creating referrals for the managed care company owned by the institution. Thus a caller is given the option, through an ACD menu, to choose English or Spanish. The subsequent ACD prompts are then given in the chosen language. The next menu presented has three choices: (1) make an appointment; (2) renew a prescription; (3) obtain a referral. If the caller chooses "Spanish" and "referral," the SBR system then looks for the next available agent who spoke Spanish and had been trained to perform referrals.

It is not always possible to completely match an available agent with high scores on the relevant criteria with the caller. This is where the SBR design becomes complicated. Also, most call centers try to minimize the time a caller spends in queue (on hold). Thus, the caller who desires to speak Spanish and request a referral may be connected with an agent who speaks Spanish but has less experience with referrals rather than being on hold until an agent who meets all of the criteria becomes available.

As the number of SBR choices increases, the design complexity can rise exponentially. It is often a long project to implement SBR so that it adds to the level of service provided by the call center. However, the rewards in efficiently and completely meeting the caller's needs can yield large benefits.

Computer Telephony Integration (CTI). CTI brings together the voice processing aspects of the call center with the existing data and systems of the institution. CTI is the marriage of the voice systems with the institution's existing systems.

Based on information collected by the voice system, CTI permits relevant information to be displayed on the agent's workstation at the same time that the call is transferred to the agent. The voice system can establish information about the caller through several means. Two of the most commonly used means of establishing who is calling are automatic number identification (ANI) and an integrated voice response (IVR) system.

ANI relies on information sent along with the phone call. ANI makes caller ID services from your local phone company possible. The ANI information includes the phone number from which the call is being placed. Information is retrieved from the call by the PBX and passed along a separate channel to the application that controls the agent's workstation. The application performs a database look-up and provides the information to the agent. The application controls the transfer of the call and the data display in a coordinated fashion. This works well when the customer calls from his or her home phone, but if the call is made from work or a pay phone, the look-up will not find a valid record. When using any form of a customer identifier to look up data, always have the agent check with the caller to ensure that the two are the same.

Whatever mode is used to collect caller identification information, the ability to provide the data access at the same time as the call is transferred significantly reduces the length of the call by eliminating the process of verbally collecting sufficient caller information for the agent to look up data. Shorter, more efficient calls benefit both the institution's customers and the institution.

Beyond the increased efficiency, CTI can also improve the ability of the call center to track when a call is received and what transpired during the call. Thus, the CTI application can automatically update the relevant patient records with the time and duration of the call, the purpose of the call, and also if there should be some follow-up activity.

Some of the information collected during the call is keyed in by the agent as prompted by the application. Many of the major healthcare information systems vendors have recognized the importance of tracking telephone interactions with patients and have provided fields in their systems for such information.

Other information collected during the call, especially if it does not actually involve an agent, such as canceling an appointment, can automatically update the relevant scheduling systems as well as trigger a follow-up action for rescheduling.

Integrated Voice Response. IVR is bringing the power of the computer to the caller through the telephone keypad or spoken word. IVR can be thought of "ACD menus all grown up" because IVR brings a level of interactivity to the caller-system interaction. When calling into a call center with an IVR, the system can request information such as the caller's identification number (e.g., patient number or social security number). With this information, the call can be more easily routed to the appropriate agent and the appropriate data will be routed along with the call through CTI. IVR is most useful when paired with CTI.

IVR technology also makes possible the self-serve model. Because the IVR is interconnected to the institution's systems, the caller can request information or complete a task without speaking with an agent. Example of interactions facilitated by an IVR in a self-serve model include the following.

- Patients can inquire when their next appointment is scheduled.
- A future appointment can be canceled.
- A prescription refill can be requested.

In all of these cases, the IVR establishes the caller's request, usually through the prompted menu system; looks up the relevant databases or accesses the relevant application; and provides information to the caller (e.g., "your next appointment is scheduled for Wednesday, 23 September 1998, with Dr. Olmsted at his Drala Avenue office") or issues an action (such as sending a refill request to the pharmacy and then providing the caller information as to when the prescription will be ready).

Enabling this level of interactivity requires great effort in creating the necessary CTI middleware, linking the systems to the IVR, and designing the appropriate prompted menu systems. The result, however, is extremely beneficial in increasing the ability of the call center to provide service to the patients, members, and other customers.

Fax on Demand (FOD). FOD is an easy addition to any call center. Through FOD, the caller can request that certain items be sent to a fax machine of their choice. Information that readily lends itself to being faxed include the following.

- Directions to the medical center, to a physician's office, or to a test facility
- Pretest preparation procedures, such as what to wear, immediate 24-hour dietary restrictions, etc.
- Physicians in a given area who are currently accepting new managed care patients

Many of these items are on standard lists maintained ready for faxing. More advanced use of FOD includes integrating the institution's systems with the FOD systems to allow faxing of unique information such as the patient's bill, recent laboratory results, discharge summaries, and any other information that the institution chooses to make available in this manner. The level of FOD requires the call center systems to properly identify and authenticate the caller before faxing. Some FOD documents may be limited to physicians who are registered in the main healthcare information system as providing care to the patient in question.

The Web-Enabled Call Center. The ability of a customer of the institution to access the call center using the World Wide Web is a new development. The entire area of Web commerce is nascent. It is possible for customers to use the Web to access some of the core call center systems and essentially view the data display.

Given the nature of healthcare data, it will require more time for the technology and the security issues to mature before the Web can be a significant addition to a healthcare institution's call center. Leading edge institutions should carefully watch electronic commerce developments to identify how the advances made can be transferred to healthcare given the semi-unique privacy requirements of healthcare as well as the need to carefully control transaction load volume of the core information systems.

It Is the People

All of the fancy and expensive technology is wasted unless the call center agents and management are up to par. Ultimately, most of the callers will be connected with an agent. These agents represent the institution every bit as much as the nurse, the physician, or the others involved in delivering and supporting patient care.

Carefully selecting agents for aptitude, attitude, and availability is crucial. Contrary to some preconceived notions, the boisterous people who are always talking may not be the best agents. Agents must have a desire to help people. Good agents like learning and have the capability to rapidly absorb new information. Good agents must be comfortable with the routine day-in, day-out process of working in a call center. Very few agents think of working at a call center as a career; it is a job.

Unlike many major call center environments which view agents as interchangeable, healthcare agents must to be thoroughly trained in the applications, in the main healthcare information systems which they access, in the institution's protocols, in special skills for areas of specialty, and in customer service. Agents need to receive consistent feedback from call center supervisors and management.

To provide proper supervision and feedback, call center supervisors should monitor calls as a quality control measure. Many healthcare institutions also record calls for training, supervision, and legal purposes. Use of monitoring tools will help call center management ascertain the productivity of the agents. Many monitoring systems will provide real-time data that can be displayed in the corner of agents' screens so that they know how they are doing also.

Call center agents have a high burnout rate. Given the training needed to have a qualified agent in a healthcare setting, turnover must be held to a minimum. Various techniques may be employed to minimize agent burnout and turnover. Table 10.2 lists some of these techniques.

Creating an ergonomic work environment is a crucial element of physical design of the call center. Information systems personnel may think primarily in terms of the computer workstation and perhaps also of objects like keyboard trays, mouse pads, and monitor stands. These are all important. Other critical ergonomic elements include lighting and noise reduction.

A roomful of people all talking on the telephone has dramatically higher requirements for noise control than does a general cubicle-based office. The headset is one of the key pieces of equipment for the agent and is not an area in which the least expensive choice should be sought.

Benefits of Call Center Technology

Benefits of call center technology may be organized into four categories: customer service, efficiency of doing business, flexibility through features and functions, and scalability. Call centers are about customer service. Customer service levels are improved by reducing the amount of time patients wait for contact with the correct representative to address the call. By reducing the amount of time spent on transferring calls and the number of times the patient contacts a representative in error, frustration levels are reduced.

In addition to reducing wait times, customer service times are reduced by having patient information available when the call is received as opposed to making the patient wait or returning the call to complete the transaction. Patients will repeat information less often and reach a successful conclusion to a call with greater frequency.

Table 10.2. Factors That Can Reduce Call Center Agent Burnout and Turnover

Ergonomic work environment
Regular breaks
Use of part-time shifts
Rotating personnel off the phone to other tasks during the day
Providing opportunities for advancement
Involvement in call center design changes
Contests and awards

By reducing wait times, service times, and increasing the frequency with which calls are brought to a successful conclusion, representatives can increase customer satisfaction rates and have a direct impact on the likelihood that a patient will use the healthcare providers and facility again.

Call centers require a great deal of up-front investment. When properly deployed, the call center can help reduce costs. However, if cost reduction is the only goal sought by an institution, there may be other avenues that it should pursue. Call centers are cost-effective means to substantially increase the quality and level of service to the institution's customers. Compared with simply staffing a large group of people to field every call, call centers are cost savers.

By reducing the frequency with which front-line clinical and administrative personnel are interrupted by phone calls to a practice, the call center can help control staffing costs and make clinical personnel more effective.

The cost of doing business may decrease with call center technology. This is a function of the impact of automating day-to-day activities, reducing the amount of time it takes to complete tasks. More efficient representatives take less time to complete individual tasks, and can, over the course of a day, respond to more calls for assistance. Management can better oversee these processes through reporting and monitoring of activity, and take action to create a more productive environment.

Call center technology can also reduce the cost of doing business with the components that reduce unnecessary traffic and eliminate the human decision-making process which can introduce errors when the knowledge base needed to make decisions is incomplete.

Flexibility is gained through the use of call center technology. Services, which once required patients to be physically present, can be deployed through the use of call centers. For example, instead of using the emergency room as a facility for nonurgent care, call center technology can by used to offer patients basic information about their illness, and then offer them possible ways to address the illness either with or without the use of healthcare professionals.

In the midst of changes with managed care, healthcare institutions can greatly improve business as well as increase revenue by offering creative services and reducing the number of unnecessary visits to their institutions. Creative services can also increase market share by offering new avenues of access to healthcare services.

Call center technology offers many options in its deployment, making it scalable in a variety of management structures. Depending on the technical infrastructure, it can support centralized or decentralized modalities, large and small environments, formal or informal settings, and single or multiple enterprises. As virtual call centers become more widely deployed, solutions not only will be scalable, but will also be dynamic, always changing to meet the particular demands of the period.

A Brief Case Study

To bring together all the elements discussed herein, a brief example follows. Kirk Heath System (KHS) is a major institution composed of three acute-care sites, plus a network of community and institution-owned ambulatory care practices. KHS implements a call center at the corporate level. KHS had several objectives for the call center, including the following.

- Reduce the time that its primary and specialty ambulatory care clinic staff spend answering the telephone because these tasks interrupt interactions with patients physically present in the clinics and often lead to many patients on the phone being put on hold.
- Eliminate the busy signal received by patients over 54 percent of the time when calling one of the ambulatory practices. This was discovered in a patient satisfaction survey and was substantiated by reviewing lost call logs from the institution's telephone system.
- Increase use of the three institution-owned pharmacies for patient prescription refills. This had the triple goal of increasing pharmacy revenue, more complete understanding of all the medications taken by a patient, and more accurately trapping prescription drug expenses for use in managed care contracting.
- Handle patient referral requests more efficiently.
- Be able to provide the right treatment, at the right location, at the right time.

To accomplish these objectives, KHS created a call center. The components included a dedicated PBX; a custom application for use by the call center agents which served as a front-end to multiple separate back-end systems (admission discharge and transfer [ADT], two laboratory systems, ambulatory information system, patient financial systems, scheduling system, pharmacy system, enterprise master person index); IVR; ACD; SBR; and FOD.

A caller to the KHS call center was greeted with a message controlled by the IVR providing the warning to call 911 if it was a medical emergency, followed by a request that the caller pick his or her language of preference. All subsequent prompts were given in the chosen language. Languages supported included English, Spanish, Russian, Vietnamese, and Tagalog, reflecting the primary populations served by KHS. Once KHS had a sufficient number of agents who spoke Mandarin, they planned to add this choice also.

A service vendor translated all of the IVR scripts to the corresponding languages, which was verified by native speakers for completeness and accuracy. The process of adding a new language took 12 weeks from beginning to end.

Once language was established, the caller was requested to type in a KHS patient identification number (KHS-ID). If this could not be verified or if the patient pressed 1 to indicate that he or she did not know the KHS-ID, other choices were presented such as social security number (SSN) and date of birth

(DOB) or home phone and DOB. Failure to locate a valid patient in the enterprise master patient index routed the caller to an agent. ANI information was captured for the call and used to attempt looking up data if the use of KHS-ID failed.

All IVR prompts provided three ways of automatically being routed to an agent: pressing zero on the telephone keypad, failing to make a choice correctly after two tries, or pressing no keys after 30 seconds.

All phones from the ambulatory clinics were rerouted to the call center. This freed the clinic personnel to concentrate their efforts on treating patients at the clinics. This alone increased the ability of the clinics to see patients by almost 10 percent. This also meant that the caller no longer received a busy signal nor was left on hold for lengthy periods, as was the case previously.

As part of the customer-focused initiative, all calls remained in a queue for an agent for no more than one minute. Through the use of the ACD and monitoring tools, supervisors and managers could jump in and field calls at peak demand times (usually Monday mornings and during lunch hours).

The caller had several choices: medical questions, appointments, prescription renewals, billing questions, speak with a representative. Callers who chose the billing option were transferred to the patient accounting department, while medical questions were transferred to the group of advice nurses.

Prescription renewals routed the caller to a series of IVR-controller menus which asked for the prescription number or attempted, through look-ups, to identify the prescription that the caller wished to renew. If the prescription did not have authorized refills, the caller was routed to an agent who would be presented with the relevant data. The agent would formulate the request to the physician for additional refill authorizations. KHS plans to add an outbound calling function to call patients and inform them when the prescription is ready.

The appointments menu choice permits the caller to check on upcoming appointments or to cancel an appointment. Requests to reschedule are routed to an agent. Appointment cancellations will, in the future, create a list for outbound calling to reschedule the appointment. Related to this, KHS also plans to begin outbound calling for appointment reminders.

For patients calling with medical questions, the call center was staffed by advice nurses. The advice nurses were logged into the system as agents in a special set of ACD queues so that they did not receive general agent calls. All calls for medical advice first went to the agents who verified the caller's demographic information and then transferred the caller to the advice nurse. When the call was transferred, the call and any relevant data were transferred to the advice nurse.

With the use of advice nurses in the call center, KHS was able to reduce inappropriate clinic visits, reduce emergency room utilization, and encourage patients to call with their questions and concerns. This enabled KHS to advance its goal of the right treatment, in the right location, at the right time.

Patients were guided toward the most appropriate treatment and because it did not entail unnecessary visits, KHS moved a step toward improving overall health management of its community.

Behind the scenes, SBR enabled KHS to route calls to agents based on language skills as well as familiarity with various clinical practices. Scheduling for some ambulatory practices involves greater complexity. Many of the outpatient dermatology surgeries involve scheduling the physician, the surgery suite, the surgery team, and the recovery room. Some agents have been trained on this complex scheduling process and therefore their skill resumé in the system would indicate this skill. Thus a Spanish-speaking patient calling for a dermatology appointment would be routed to an agent with the appropriate skill.

To get the call center off the ground, KHS offered many of the clinic front-desk staff positions in the call center. This enabled KHS to create a call center with agents who were familiar with the environment and procedures. As new agents are hired they are run through a tour of duty within the clinics to make them familiar with KHS. Some agents divide their work time between the clinics and the call center. This helps agents maintain their ties to the practices as well as reduce some of the burnout associated with full-time call center work.

The KHS call center is still being refined. To date, the cost of the call center has exceeded several million dollars. The primary benefits to date have come in the areas of improved patient satisfaction, improved clinic operations, and reduced clinic staff growth.

The Future

Call centers have much to offer healthcare in terms of improving customer satisfaction, enabling new initiatives, controlling costs, and enhancing collections. Call centers are a combination of technology and people which link together the resources of the organization in support of the institution's goals.

In this article, we have dealt with a number of areas of the call center. Institutions that desire to pursue the benefits of call centers must create a team to investigate and manage the process. The team must include clinical, administrative, telephony, and information systems personnel because the call center crosses many organizational boundaries. Outside expert help can often make the difference between success and failure for large call center projects.

Suggested Readings

Benson B. New hospital phone technology allows patients to call in sick. *Crain's New York Business.* October 2, 1995:14.
Bozeman M. Why aren't call centers doing better? *TeleProfessional.* June 1996:22–30.
Dawson K. The benefits of a virtual call center. Quicklink.com/dawson/virtual.htm.
Grandinetti D. Patient phone calls driving you crazy? *Med Econ.* June 24, 1996:72–88.
Karve A. Operator, give me telephony. *LAN Mag.* July 1994:71–77.

Luongo J. The five most important questions to ask help desk software vendors. *Teleprofessional.* March 1996:24–28.

State of the Union: US call centers in 1996. Vanguard.net/vanguard/state/html.

About the Authors

Gerard M. Nussbaum, MS, CPA, CMA, RCDD, is a senior manager with Hamilton HMC.

Star P. Ault, MS, MBA, is a manager with Hamilton HMC.

Providence Health Plan Call Center: A Case Study in Innovation and Integration

Miriam Odermann; Gregory J. Petras; Janeen Cook

The harsh realities facing the healthcare system in America in the waning years of the millennium have created both confusion and clarity among healthcare providers, consumers, and insurers. The introduction of managed care and capitation and the rise of health maintenance organizations (HMOs) has initiated a vast sea of change, moving healthcare from being a fragmented industry with few controls and little accountability to one in which control and accountability set the foundation. As payers have reduced reimbursements, it has become apparent that healthcare providers have to be proactive in managing care to better manage costs. They have been challenged to reduce costs and improve outcomes.

To achieve both objectives, providers are changing the ways in which healthcare is delivered, moving from a reactive mode, in which the focus is on treating illness, to a proactive mode, in which the focus is on maintaining health and wellness. A healthy, active population is less likely to burden the healthcare system in the years to come, particularly that anomalous segment known as the baby boomers, who, in significant numbers, are now moving into middle age.

The healthcare industry has realized that, in this environment, the joint challenges of achieving cost containment and effecting positive outcomes can be met only through the deployment of electronic and automated technologies that process and network relevant data. Many such technologies are being used in applications such as telephony and voice systems used in hospital or clinic medical call centers. To encourage the use of appropriate clinical resources offered through the healthcare organization, the provider may choose to use a call center thus increasing the number of customers it serves and enhancing customer communication, service, and loyalty.

In the past, medical call centers have been used primarily as marketing tools to increase a healthcare organization's identity awareness and visibility in highly competitive markets. In most of these cases, the call center was operated independently from the healthcare organization and provided services such as physician referrals, 24-hour triage and advice, and automated health information.

But as call centers become an integral part of the care delivery process, it is imperative that they become an integrated spoke on the "enterprise wheel" with access to the same information as other points of care. Integrating a call center's services with a database networking system would serve a much larger and geographically dispersed health plan member population and help the provider achieve the dual objectives of lowering costs and improving outcomes.

Background

Providence Health System of Portland, Oregon, envisioned such a system. Five years ago, Providence made the decision to migrate from the traditional healthcare model to an integrated delivery system based on managed care and cost containment. In 1995, the organization began implementing the necessary components to achieve a fully integrated data environment that would proactively serve its members and keep its healthcare costs at a minimum. Providence currently manages 25 acute care facilities in the states of Oregon and California as well as a home health service in Oregon and a managed care insurance organization called the Providence Health Plan.

The goal of the organization in all its operations is to provide "seamless access" to healthcare for its more than 190,000 health plan members through the application of a comprehensive access management strategy. Such a strategy enables Providence to arrange for care by providing a consistent, coordinated process for managing member access to health services.

To streamline its operations, Providence uses the information systems, network management, and healthcare database products and services from Atlanta-based HBOC, a top provider in the healthcare informatics industry. In 1997, HBOC acquired National Health Enhancement Systems (NHES), an industry leader in medical call center technology and expertise which supports 500 installed call centers across the United States. As part of HBOC, NHES technologies and services now support one of the most crucial tactical components of Providence's strategy: a nurse triage call center to complement Providence Health Plan's automated information line, which only offers member service information.

Providence implemented the triage call center for its health plan members in January 1995 to improve access to healthcare and decrease inappropriate utilization of healthcare services. Providence quickly discovered that the call center was a tremendous asset in its integrated delivery strategy, providing a range of services to at-risk members and, at the same time, reducing the burden on physicians in the health plan. Today, Providence's call center is used by 20 percent of its health plan members annually and is differentiated from other stand-alone facility-based call centers because of the critical role it plays in Providence's integrated access management strategy.

Four Distinct Services

Since 1995, the Providence call center has expanded to offer four distinct services to the organization's health plan members.

- The Providence "RN Line" is staffed by licensed registered nurses and provides online support for members requiring medical triage and advice. It also serves as an interface with the other three services.
- The Providence AudioLibrary offers an automated reference library for information on more than 1000 healthcare topics. The reference material helps health plan members as well as the community learn more about health-related concerns and potentially assists them in making decisions about their own healthcare.
- The Providence Resource Line, staffed by resource specialists, provides assistance to health plan members and the community with selecting a primary care physician (PCP), provides information and referral to Providence Health System services and programs, and provides information and registration assistance for a health education class sponsored by Providence.
- The Care Management Line takes calls from PCPs and other healthcare providers seeking a care manager for one of their patients or to arrange for resources such as skilled nursing facility placements for patients with complex needs.

The Providence RN Line, the Resource Line, and the AudioLibrary use HBOC's Centramax M Plus and Voicemax Plus integrated database software and voice technologies. Centramax M Plus is a Windows-based software system that applies clinically tested adult and pediatric algorithms to provide appropriate care and time-related triage to callers in the most cost-effective setting. Using a dedicated server, the system runs as a stand-alone network. The software is compliant with HL7 (Health Level 7) and can therefore transfer data from one healthcare entity to another. Voicemax Plus uses voice-response technology to integrate with a user's telephone system. It offers members access to healthcare information by touch telephone, 24 hours a day, seven days a week.

For database and network management of its health plan, Providence uses HBOC's AMISYS 3000 information system. Currently, Providence staff members download member information from the AMISYS 3000 database twice a month to keep the RN Line database up to date. In the future, integration between the two systems will enable call center staff to access full medical histories online as well as add to the records with each call, thereby creating a more robust information database at the nurses' disposal.

RN Line

Using Providence's database of demographic information on health plan members, the RN Line's objectives are to increase member satisfaction with access to healthcare through Providence and to decrease unnecessary emergency room utilization and inappropriate physician office visits. The RN Line functions as a gateway to healthcare services, providing medical advice as well as promoting wellness behavior, improving consumer and physician satisfaction, reducing costs, and improving consumer access to healthcare resources.

The Providence RN lines are staffed by licensed RNs who respond to a caller's healthcare needs with a combination of customized software, clinical guidelines approved by the Providence RN Physician Advisory Committee, and professional judgment. Members calling into the RN Line are presented with a message instructing them to hang up and dial 911 if it is a medical emergency; otherwise they are instructed to hold for the next available RN, and after 30 seconds they have the opportunity to leave a voicemail message for an RN to call them back.

As the calls are routed to an RN, a call display feature alerts the RN with caller identification based on the number the caller dialed to reach the RN. Using the Centramax M Plus program with its symptom-based guidelines (frequently updated with new medical information), the RN queries the caller to ascertain the level of urgency. Clusters of questions move from "most acute" to "least acute" as the RN is directed through the triage guidelines to a recommended course of action. The RN, depending on the type and severity of the symptom, will offer specific advice to the caller on how to deal with the situation.

Disposition of the call can vary from an RN assisting the member to contact his or her PCP within 15 minutes in a case requiring urgent care, to an RN providing instruction on how to alleviate the patient's symptoms at home in a case without need for medical care. Following a call, the member's PCP receives a fax from the call center informing him or her of the patient's call, the RN's recommended action, and the final disposition of the situation. All calls are reported in this way to the member's PCP to keep the personal physician involved. (Even in an emergency situation, the call center would only send the member to an emergency room if the RN was unable to reach the PCP within the recommended time frame.)

The average call, including "talk" and "computer time," ranges from 10 to 12 minutes. On-screen material is readily available at every RN workstation through the Centramax M Plus software. When on the line with a caller, the RN can also exit from the Centramax M Plus software with the member's on-screen file and then access the AMISYS 3000 system for additional information. Providence plans to integrate all systems so that the information available from the AMISYS 3000 database is accessible online during a call, without having to exit from the Centramax system.

The RN Line also functions in a proactive capacity by having RNs make outbound calls to follow up on health plan members who have visited an emergency department within the previous 24 hours for a nonemergency medical concern. The database collects information on a member from various sources, then synthesizes the data, and makes it available in a single file.

For example, information in the database file might indicate that a member suffers from a chronic illness such as diabetes or asthma. The RN would call the member according to information on file in the database and ensure that the patient is adhering to his or her physician's instructions. This can prevent problems from arising or from escalating to a crisis and thereby reduce costly healthcare visits.

After Hours Call Support

In addition to fielding calls from Providence members, Portland area physicians have contracted with Providence to provide after hours call support through its call center. The call center does not serve as an answering service but rather functions as an extension of the PCP's office. When answering service personnel receive a call from a patient or customer, they report it to the Providence RN Line and leave a message on voicemail. RN Line staff members check the line's voicemail and return the PCP office calls promptly.

RNs work staggered hours, staffing up during the peak hours of 7 to 9 AM, lunch hour, after work, and in the evening hours. They also increase staff numbers for peak times during the year, such as flu and cold season, using on-call RNs to fill in as required. The ratio for adequate staffing has proven to be one full-time equivalent RN for approximately 8000 calls annually. Providence is experimenting with some RNs working out of their homes using laptops and dedicated telephone lines.

Benefits

The Inter-Hospital Physician Association (IPA), whose goal is population health improvement, funds the Providence call center. Health plan members who use the service are not billed for its use, nor does usage affect the cost of their premiums.

Today Providence call center provides benefits to health plan members and their physicians and to Providence itself by improving patient access to medical care and information. Customer satisfaction, and therefore customer loyalty, is enhanced. Call center usage contributes to the building of robust patient database profiles, while reducing the costs of care and minimizing the burden on physician offices, clinics, and hospitals. Finally, the call center markets the Providence Health Plan to a larger community and to potential customers.

Providence has established a solid foundation for its vision of seamless access through the strategic deployment of electronic and automated technologies. The organization continues to work closely with HBOC to integrate the RN Line records with the AMISYS 3000 database, merging information on all care encounters. Providence also plans to convert to a new file server called B-trieve to provide a true client/server environment, which translates to more stable, reliable data management.

Providence is looking at possibilities in its system to centralize telephone access for its members using one number to provide all services, thereby enhancing member satisfaction from triage, information, and referrals to claims data and billing records.

Conclusion

Providence is further considering the possibility of expanding the call center services outside its geographic mandate. Many are asking the question: Is providing healthcare services limited to the community or municipality served by a specific facility? To what extent can it be centralized through the use of call centers and provided to a geographically dispersed population to achieve economies of scale? Providence is pondering this issue as it evaluates the efficiency and effectiveness of its current system, leading the organization into the third millennium, and closer to realizing its vision of seamless access.

About the Authors

Miriam Odermann is Director of Outreach Services of Providence Health System in Portland, Oregon.

Gregory J. Petras is Senior Vice President and General Manager of HBOC Call Center Group in Phoenix, Arizona.

Janeen Cook is Vice President of Product Marketing of HBOC's Community Access Strategies in Atlanta.

Customer Service Call Center Infrastructure Redesign

Stephen Pratt; Jeffrey Johnson

Client Background

Late in 1994, Deloitte Consulting was brought in to conduct a major corporate reengineering project for Blue Shield of California. As part of this project, it was determined that the Blue Shield customer service call center infrastructure would require significant redesign.

Before Deloitte Consulting's involvement with Blue Shield, the environment was characterized by flat membership growth, high administrative costs, inconsistent service delivery processes and performance levels, and an inefficient call center delivery platform. The rapidly changing healthcare industry and the intensifying competition only exacerbated these internal challenges faced by Blue Shield. To effectively address both the challenges of the internal environment and the competitive pressures of the external environment, it was decided to focus on the company's ability to address varying customer service needs by providing more ways to access a broader range of information and to make it substantially easier to receive customer service from Blue Shield. Blue Shield saw a clear correlation between flexible, responsive customer service and competitive strength. In partnership with Deloitte Consulting, Blue Shield began the extensive redesign of the customer service call center infrastructure and processes.

Given the scope of reengineering at Blue Shield, it would be necessary for the customer service call center infrastructure team to work closely with members of other reengineering initiatives to understand business requirements, identify training requirements, provide support for human resource redesign efforts, and change management activities. These other reengineering efforts included Deloitte Consulting practitioners, Blue Shield employees, other consultants, and a number of Blue Shield's vendors.

Project Charter and Background Summary

The customer service call center project was kicked off in December 1994 and completed in Spring 1996. At the outset, the following specific objectives were identified.

- Create a customer-focused service environment
- Significantly improve cost-effectiveness
- Improve market responsiveness
- Reduce transaction cycle times
- Create a culture of learning and accountability

To achieve these objectives, it would be necessary to implement new call center technologies, including interactive voice response (IVR), computer telephony integration (CTI), and advanced voice network features. There were additional benefits to be gained from improving operational efficiencies.

Implementation of the IVR, CTI, and advanced voice network features would address the first four objectives. These technologies would create a greater degree of customer focus by providing Blue Shield's approximately 1.5 million member base with more options to retrieve important membership information. By providing more options, the specific needs of individual groups within the membership base would receive more focused attention. Cost-effectiveness would be improved by replacing some of the call center agents with these technologies. Market responsiveness would improve with the use of these technologies because of their ability to operate seven days per week, 24 hours per day in multiple languages. The automated nature of CTI "screen pops" in particular would reduce transaction times by eliminating precious seconds from each call. Lastly, the size and scope of the project provided an excellent opportunity to address the last objective by altering Blue Shield's call center culture to one of learning and accountability. The fundamental changes to core processes allowed Blue Shield employees to take an active role in shaping their work environment.

The project was divided into multiple phases to accommodate its large scale. Figure 12.1 shows the approximate duration of each phase. The following is a description of these phases.

Organize and Prepare the Project Team. The primary tasks included in this phase were defining the project structure and approach, identifying roles and responsibilities, and preparing the team for upcoming analysis and implementation activities. No specific project "deliverables" were produced in this phase. However, a robust project reporting structure and an organized, cohesive team were developed for the project duration.

Develop Project Work Plan and Milestones. This phase involved the following tasks: definition and communication of the project scope; development of a comprehensive project work plan; securing commitments to targeted milestones; identification of project interdependencies and critical path activities. From this phase, a project work plan was created as a project deliverable. The project work plan was then presented to Blue Shield management.

Development of Future Call Center Design. The primary tasks during this phase were to identify Blue Shield's business requirements; assist the

Figure 12.1. Call Center Transformation Project Overview

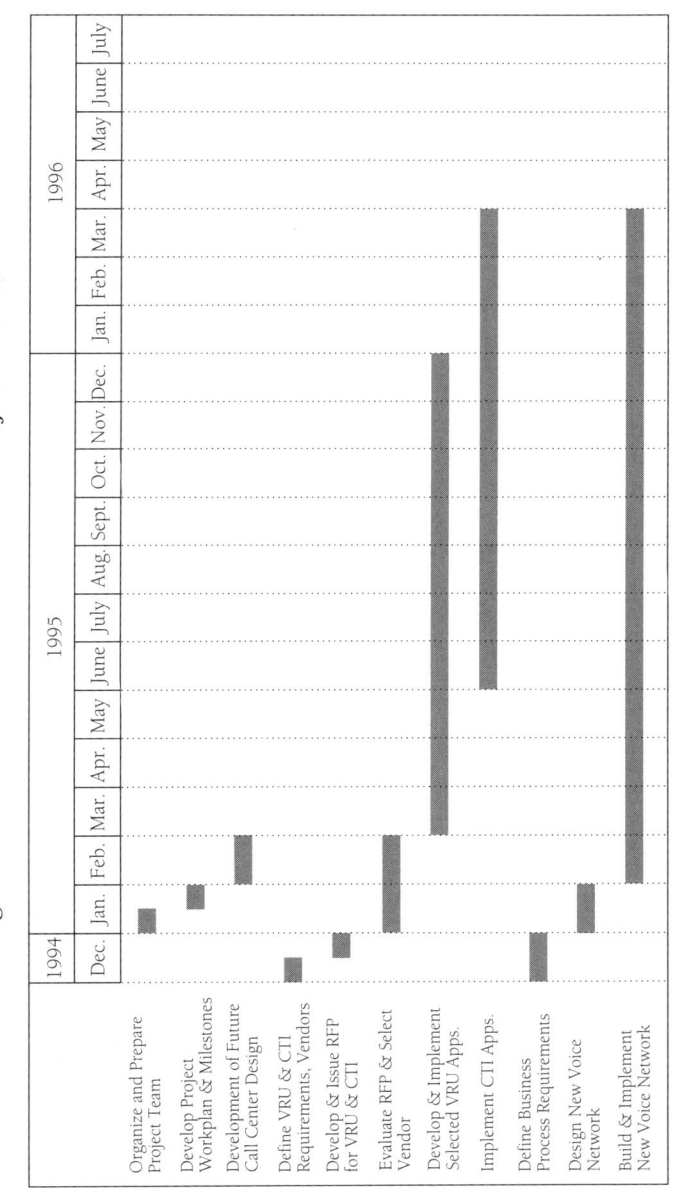

process redesign team in defining call/work flows; review marketing analysis of customer's expectations; analyze technological infrastructure requirements; develop call center network design and configuration; and validate and obtain "buy-in" for network design and call flows. Key project deliverables from this phase included definition and documentation of Blue Shield's business requirements; process maps and diagrams; analysis and documentation of customer and user expectations; identification of technical and organizational requirements; call center network and physical seating design and architecture plan; and call flow diagrams.

Define VRU and CTI Requirements and Vendors. During this phase, the following activities were undertaken: identification of Blue Shield requirements for VRU and CTI technology; analysis of existing call traffic and estimation of potential savings from VRU and CTI; analysis of VRU and CTI vendors and development of a list of targeted vendors; and comparison of vendors' VRU and CTI products. Key project deliverables created during this phase included identification of targeted VRU and CTI applications; list of potential vendors; detailed traffic analysis; and estimated savings from VRU and CTI technology implementation.

Develop and Issue a Request for Proposal (RFP) for VRU and CTI. The relevant tasks during this phase were to develop appropriate structure and format for RFP; draft the RFP; conduct validation sessions with customer service groups; develop functional and technical VRU and CTI requirements; develop target list of applications and estimate availability dates; develop preliminary call center architecture for VRU and CTI deployment; obtain management sign-off on RFP; and issue the RFP. Deliverables created during this phase included identification and documentation of targeted VRU applications for a preliminary call center architecture and design. An additional important component of this phase was to secure buy-in from Blue Shield management on the call center architecture and design and VRU and CTI applications. Finally, the RFPs for VRU and CTI are issued during this phase.

Evaluate RFP and Select Vendor. Evaluation of the RFP required the following tasks to be completed: the development of RFP evaluation criteria and scoring methodology; analysis of responses to the RFP; development of business case; selection of a preliminary winning bid; presentation of finding to Blue Shield management and obtaining concurrence; notification of selected vendor; and contract negotiation. Key deliverables from this phase included the RFP evaluation criteria, scoring methodology, and business case. During this phase the response to the RFP was communicated to Blue Shield management.

Develop and Implement Selected VRU Applications. The primary tasks during this phase were to participate in the development of required VRU menu trees; identify and understand call flows for targeted applications; conduct joint application development sessions; work with the selected vendor to develop applications; participate in the development of VRU applications and testing; define requirements for integrating the VRU with the G3I PBXs; develop implementation timeline for VRU applications; identify necessary training requirements; work with Blue Shield's marketing department to develop VRU marketing plan; roll-out selected VRU functions to Blue Shield's customers. Deliverables created during this phase included detailed call center flows and menu trees for targeted application; a detailed training plan for technical staff and others; and a VRU roll-out plan that included how the functions would be advertised to Blue Shield members. During this phase, the VRU hardware is implemented and the selected VRU applications for customer service, medical management, and membership installation were implemented.

Implement CTI Applications. The primary tasks during this phase were to participate in the development of required CTI applications; identify and understand call flows for targeted applications; conduct joint application development sessions; work with the selected vendor to develop applications; participate in the development of CTI applications and testing; develop implementation timeline for CTI applications; identify necessary training requirements; work with Blue Shield's marketing department to develop a CTI marketing plan; roll-out selected CTI functions to Blue Shield's customers. Deliverables created during this phase included detailed call center flows and menu trees for targeted application; a detailed training plan for technical staff and others; and a CTI roll-out plan that included how the functions would be advertised to Blue Shield members. During this phase, the CTI hardware was implemented and the selected CTI applications were implemented.

Define Business Process Requirements. The primary tasks during this phase were to identify Blue Shield business process requirements and future call flows; analyze call traffic; analyze and estimate future staffing and trunk requirements; and identify toll-free numbers to be consolidated. Accomplishments included call center traffic analysis and estimated staffing and trunk requirements. A list of toll-free numbers to be consolidated was created as an important project deliverable from this phase.

Design New Voice Network. During this phase, design sessions with users and vendors were conducted; the call center design was validated along with an estimate of the network cost. The design was then presented to Blue Shield management to obtain buy-in. The validated network design and the network cost estimate were important project deliverables from this phase.

Build and Implement New Voice Network. The primary tasks during this phase were to procure necessary services and hardware; develop call traffic migration and consolidation plans; assist the process team in developing the future customer interface and toll-free number strategy; manage vendor installation and/or "cutover" of new services and hardware; assist in contract negotiations; supervise the consolidation of call centers; integrate the new network with the VRU and CTI applications. The end of this phase was signified by integrating operational call center functions in the four locations. Project deliverables from this phase included negotiated contracts for related voice network services and equipment and a proposed customer interface and toll-free number strategy.

Project Scope

The Blue Shield customer service call center project began by reducing 16 service delivery sites down to 4 sites. From these 16 service delivery sites, Blue Shield supported its 1.5 million members by taking over 12 million calls per year.

To support ongoing operations, specific project assumptions were made at the beginning of the project. As new information was received, these assumptions were modified.

VRU Assumptions. There were some lines of business that would not use the VRU technology at all, while other lines of business would not use the VRU until later phases. All Blue Shield employees would be routed through the VRU and all customer service calls other than the exceptions mentioned before were to be answered by the VRU. In some cases, the VRU was either unable to support the specific needs of a particular business line or it was determined that the VRU would not provide an appropriate level of service.

CTI Assumptions. As with the VRU, some lines of business would not use the CTI technology at all and other lines of business would not use CTI until later phases. Calls transferred outside the region would not have CTI and some calls within the region would use CTI for the initial implementation. Lastly, screens were to be popped only if the call center agent was in an idle state.

Toll-Free Number Assumptions. Assumptions regarding toll-free numbers were largely based on either a need to identify a specific line of business by using a unique toll-free number or the necessity to provide a large account with its own toll-free numbers. Toll-free numbers would not be changed until the consolidation. There will be one Spanish toll-free number.

Call Routing Assumptions. Certain call routing assumptions were made; for instance, callers would be transferred to the appropriate queues based on the toll-free number they dialed and calls not being routed through the VRU would have dedicated queues.

Project Results

The primary purpose of this project was to make Blue Shield more competitive by improving customer retention; facilitating the acquisition of new individual and group accounts; securing and solidifying relationships with healthcare providers; and controlling costs.

This project produced various planned and unplanned benefits for a wide range of constituencies. Planned benefits included improved service quality, cost-effectiveness, and competitiveness, thus making this a very successful project for Blue Shield.

In spite of intensifying competition in California's healthcare insurance marketplace, Blue Shield's membership base has grown since project completion. This growth has been facilitated by a 25 percent increase in customer service quality as measured by customer surveys. Furthermore, administrative costs of healthcare have declined substantially due, in large part, to millions of dollars in recurring cost savings facilitated by applying technology to redesigned business processes.

Focusing People on "High Value" Work. One of the project's key benefits is the automation of Blue Shield's most basic customer service transactions. Customer service calls regarding eligibility, copayments, physician information, mailing addresses, or the status of a claim can be completed by the automated system without the involvement of a customer service agent. This allows Blue Shield's employees to focus on the customer transactions in which they add the most value, such as inquiries that require judgment, compassion, detailed explanations, and special handling. A marked reduction in the number of times agents manually retrieve information from databases and relay it to customers allows them to focus more on value-added customer service and less on clerical tasks. Moreover, improvements made to agent workstations allow people to be customer service experts rather than database technicians. This leads to more satisfied employees and customers.

Another key benefit of the system is that it reduces the amount of clerical work and repetition associated with transactions that reach a customer service agent. If a caller "opts out" to speak to an agent after having entered his or her social security number, the relevant policy information will be automatically "popped" to the screen of the agent as the call arrives. This allows the agent to greet the caller by his or her name and the caller does not have to repeat information. Because the agent has instant access to the caller's information, little time is wasted on clerical tasks and database searches.

Access to a Broader Range of Tailored Information. Automated access to information is not new. What is unique, however, is the scope and depth of information provided by Blue Shield's automated system. Rather than provide standardized messages designed for all members, Blue Shield's interactive system retrieves tailored information based directly on a caller's input. For example, a customer calling about a claim enters his or her social security number and the approximate date of the claim, and the system responds with the immediate status of the claim. This is in sharp contrast to more traditional systems which simply provide recorded messages telling members that claims are generally processed in three weeks. This access method is not only simple and quick, but also conforms to federally mandated guidelines related to customer privacy.

Flexible Access to Information. Automated access in and of itself is not sufficient; people have substantially different needs and preferences when it comes to customer service. Accordingly a key component of Blue Shield's customer service delivery system is its flexibility.

First and foremost, customers do not have to use the automated system during business hours; that is, they are given the option of using it. Those who choose to use it can "opt out" at any time to speak with an agent. While we would like to think that everyone appreciates the virtues of the system, the simple fact is that many people would much rather receive "human" service. As people become more accustomed to automated service, we expect to see a rise in the proportion of people who complete their entire transactions within the system.

Second, the interactive system has been developed in both English and Spanish to account for the fact that 30 percent of California's population prefers or is reliant on the Spanish language. The Asian community is the second largest ethnic group in California and is growing rapidly; therefore a future phase of the system's implementation will likely include the addition of Cantonese.

Third, the automated system's operating hours are not limited to those of the customer service staff. While extended hours staffing is currently not cost-effective, the automated system can provide a fairly broad range of after-hours service.

Finally, the system is flexible enough to account for the fact that people do not always have all the information related to their transaction. For example, callers checking on the status of a claim do not need to know the exact date of their medical service. Once a customer enters an approximate date, the system locates the most likely claim.

Reduced Administrative Load for Medical Care Providers. Another beneficiary of the automated system is California's healthcare provider community. When our members visit care providers, the provider's administrative staff must verify patient eligibility with Blue Shield. Using the patient's membership card and Blue Shield's automated system, the administrative staff members can quickly verify coverage and turn their focus to providing medical care. In fact, some of these administrative staff members are so proficient at using the automated system that they do not wait for the prompts—they have memorized the key patterns. Healthcare providers are usually affiliated with multiple health plans, of which Blue Shield is but one. The administrative staff often have strong opinions about the plans and frequently provide advice to patients. The more satisfied they are with the service they receive, the more likely they are to refer potential members to Blue Shield.

Increased Availability of Healthcare Coverage. Increased operating efficiency has enabled Blue Shield to decrease the price of its individual family plan coverage. By decreasing the price of this plan, which is targeted at individuals and families who do not have coverage through large employers, Blue Shield has expanded its enrollment among a population that has traditionally had less access to healthcare insurance. The operational efficiencies that have made it possible to be profitable at lower rates were enabled by the successful implementation of the technologies described herein.

Broader Societal Benefits. While the benefits outlined here were planned and deliberate, there are a number of additional benefits that are natural by-products of our project. The additional benefits detailed below became apparent as Blue Shield progressed through project implementation.

New Standards for Service. By raising customer service standards, Blue Shield is leading the development of customer orientation within the historically unresponsive healthcare insurance industry. While many in our industry have focused on acquiring membership bases through mergers and acquisitions, our efforts have raised consumer expectations and helped establish customer service as a basis for effective competition.

New Models for Cooperation. This project brought together and leveraged the expertise of a broad range of internal and external resources. In total, the project involved two internal technology groups, more than three operational units, several marketing groups, five leading-edge technology vendors, and a leading consulting firm. The models for interaction and cooperation developed during this project will surely help both Blue Shield and its partners implement other successful projects in the future.

New Vendor Capabilities. At the commencement of this project, the capabilities for completion simply did not exist. The progress made by and between vendors during the implementation of this project will likely pave the way for advancements both within and outside our industry.

Project Technical Specifications

The technical plan called for an integrated infrastructure supporting four primary call centers located in geographically dispersed sites (Figure 12.2). Both IVR and CTI technologies support the call centers. The VRU was supplied by Periphonics and the CTI was supplied by Lucent.

Project Time Frame

Overall, the project took 16 months. Vendor management, staff shortages, and technology challenges led to project delays throughout the duration of the project. Vendor delays occurred because of difficulties in obtaining full vendor support during intensive parts of the project. Staff shortages were also a source of delay. There were times during the project when the volume of work exceeded the client's capacity to complete it. In those cases, it was necessary to hire additional resources. Delays due to technology challenges were also encountered. The complexity of the technology and the lack of a large installed base required the team to overcome multiple challenges that would normally have been avoided if more mature technologies existed. As solutions were developed for these problems, it was sometimes necessary to adjust the project schedule.

Figure 12.2. Technical Infrastructure Supporting Four Geographically Dispersed Call Centers

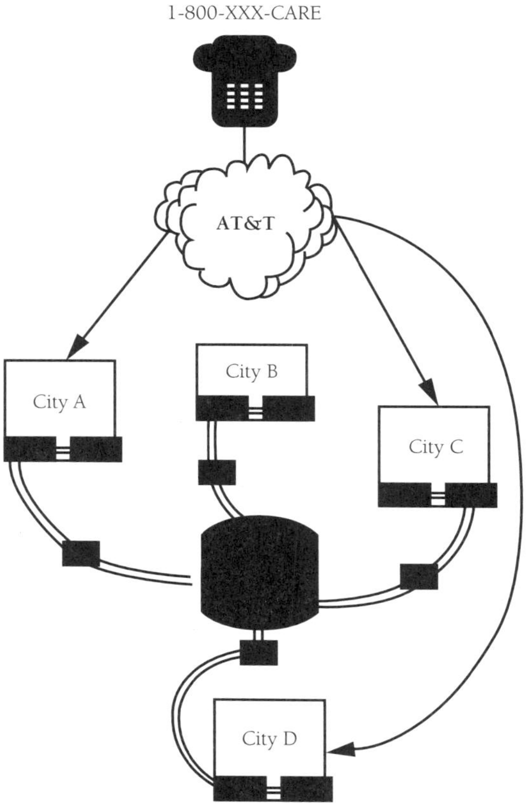

Project Risks and Risk Mitigation

Over the course of the project, the team encountered multiple risks, including technology adoption, vendor management, team morale, and communication. The impact of these risks was, most often, a delay in the project.

Although Blue Shield had implemented complex technologies in the past, they were largely relegated to back-office functions and therefore did not have broad-reaching impact. The IVR and CTI technologies being implemented in the customer service call center project were more complex than most and pervaded throughout the organization and beyond to Blue Shield's membership base.

The complexity and newness of these technologies created a high degree of risk associated with their adoption. This risk had to be managed within the

Blue Shield operating environment and the membership base. Within the Blue Shield operating environment, the call center managers and staff were required to accept new processes for performing their jobs, with a more extensive involvement with technology than they were accustomed to. For example, the use of CTI "screen pops" was an entirely new method of approaching member communications. To overcome the risk in this area extensive training was required at all levels: the call center agent, the supervisor, and the manager. The approach to training was based on developing a common base of knowledge pertaining to the technology being implemented rather than attempting to hide the technical aspects of the technology. A series of "dog and pony shows" were developed to communicate and build a better understanding of the technology.

Risk associated with vendor management required constant vigilance throughout the project, particularly toward the end of the project when deadlines were approaching, technologies were becoming operational, and team fatigue was at a maximum. The risk was greatest when vendor-related problems arose which had not been anticipated and problems were not always clear. At these times, the vendors were often asked to go to great lengths to overcome problems which were characteristically resisted, thus jeopardizing project deadlines. At the core of managing vendor risk was planning. During the early stages of the project, detailed plans were assembled which addressed technical, operational, and human resource issues. In addition, a rigorous RFP process was undertaken to fully understand vendor capabilities and their fit with Blue Shield's requirements. Sweating the details at the beginning of the project alleviated much of the pain at the end of the project.

Team morale was an important source of risk throughout the project. The project team was made up of many members: consultants, clients, vendors, and end users. The project work environment was often one of long hours and tight deadlines. As such, it was necessary for project managers to continually gauge the team's morale. The downside of low morale was burn-out which would lead to mistakes in the workplace and, in the worst-case scenario, accidents that could potentially be harmful to the team members themselves. Managing risk of this kind involved recognizing the signs of loss of morale and burn-out and then taking steps to counter it. These steps included off-site events for team building, celebrations when milestones were reached, and recognition of superior efforts on the job.

On projects of this size and scope, there is a great need for communication because the actions of one part of a team are likely to affect not only the rest of that team but also the efforts of other project teams. Furthermore, there is a substantial risk associated with the communication of false information. During the course of the customer service call center project, there were times when false information was communicated. In some cases, this caused substantial delays, particularly when actions had been taken based on false information. During this project, it was necessary to develop a structured approach to communications on many projects; this is part of an overall communications plan. For example, from the project outset, weekly meetings were scheduled to ensure not only that basic project information was being communicated but also that tasks were being accomplished and that all team members were aware of what their colleagues were doing. Through these meetings, major and minor issues were addressed and solutions developed.

Client Satisfaction

Based on this project, Blue Shield of California received the Smithsonian Institution's finalist medal for innovative use of technology. The results of this project have exceeded Blue Shield's expectations and continue to provide lasting returns to the organization.

About the Authors

Stephen Pratt is the Global Leader of Deloitte & Touche Consulting Group's Customer Dynamics Service Line.

Jeffrey Johnson is a manager in the Deloitte & Touche Consulting Group's San Francisco office.

HIMSS RESOURCES

To order: Contact HIMSS, (312) 664-HIMSS (4467); web site: http://www.himss.org; or fax on demand: 1-800-HIMSS-11 (1-800-446-7711). Also contact HIMSS for more information about additional HIMSS resources for the health care information and management systems professional.

Books

Work Study for Hospitals is a guide for those who practice hospital work sampling or manage staff or consultants in this field. Composed of 22 chapters, 71 figures, and 240 pages.
Price: HIMSS members, $38; nonmembers, $50

Guide to Effective Health Care Clinical Systems provides an introduction and overview of clinical systems for professionals in clinical and information systems, management engineering, and telecommunications. 80 pages.
Price: HIMSS members $10; non-members $15
(Volume discounts available on 25 or more)

Guide to Effective Health Care Telecommunications discusses the role and organization of telecommunications management including an historical perspective, strategic planning, enabling technologies, and needs analysis. 140 pages.
Price: HIMSS members $10; non-members $15
(Volume discounts available on 25 or more)

Guide to Effective Health Care Management Engineering explains the crucial role of the management engineer in health care today, and presents the tools and techniques that make the management engineer a critical team member. 34 pages.
Price: HIMSS members $10; non-members $15
(Volume discounts available on 25 or more)

Guide to Nursing Informatics provides a glossary of terms and key concepts that can be used as preparation for the American Nurses' Credentialing Center (ANCC) certification exam or as a reference for practicing nurses.
Price: HIMSS members $10; non-members $15
(Volume discounts available on 25 or more)

Conference Proceedings

Proceedings of the 1998 Annual HIMSS Conference and Exhibition (Orlando, FL), 4-volume boxed set, approximately 1,500 pages, 157 educational sessions, and 36 poster presentations.
Price: HIMSS members $65; non-members $95

CD-ROM/Proceedings of the 1998 Annual HIMSS Conference and Exhibition (Orlando, FL), fully searchable/retrievable text and graphics of the technical presentations, attendee roster, and poster presentation. Bonus! The Proceedings of the 1997 Annual Conference and Exhibition (San Diego, CA), and results of the '95, '96, and '97 Annual HIMSS Leadership Surveys.
Price: HIMSS members $90; non-members $135

Proceedings of the 1997 Annual HIMSS Conference and Exhibition (San Diego, CA), 4-volume boxed set, approximately 1,500 pages, 140 educational sessions, and 17 poster presentations.
Price: HIMSS members $45; non-members $65

CD-ROM/Proceedings of the 1996 Annual HIMSS Conference and Exhibition (Atlanta, GA), fully searchable/retrievable text and graphics, 88 educational sessions, and 14 poster presentations.
Price: HIMSS members $65; non-members $95

Audio/Visual

Sessions for all HIMSS educational events are available from ACTS INC., (314)394-0611, fax (314)394-9381.

Healthcare Information and Management Systems Society

The Healthcare Information and Management Systems Society (HIMSS) provides leadership in health care for the management of systems, information, and change. Its 10,000 professional members include individuals in the fields of clinical systems, information systems, management engineering, and telecommunications working in health care organizations throughout the world and dedicated to promoting a better understanding of health care information and management systems.

HIMSS performs and publishes research in key areas including the HIMSS Annual Leadership Survey on trends in health care computing and the Annual HIMSS Compensation Study. In addition, HIMSS sponsors the most comprehensive annual conference and exhibition in this field, as well as numerous regional educational events.

For more information about membership, publications, and educational events, contact HIMSS at 312/664–HIMSS (4467), Web Site: http://www.himss.org, E-mail: himss@himss.org, or Fax-on-Demand Service: 800/HIMSS–11 (800/446–7711).

1997–1998 HIMSS Officers

President
Cynthia Spurr, MBA, RNC, FHIMSS, Corporate Director, Clinical Systems Management, Partners HealthCare System, Boston, MA

Vice President
Cherryl Turner, FHIMSS, Project Leader, HBO & Company, Atlanta, GA

President-Elect
Jeffrey Cooper, FHIMSS, Vice President, Ancillary Services and CIO, Henry Medical Center, Stockbridge, GA

Vice President-Elect
Pamela Matthews, FHIMSS, Senior Consultant, KPMG Peat Marwick, LLP, Atlanta, GA

1997–1998 HIMSS Directors

Nancy Aldrich, FHIMSS, President, Telecommunications Management Corporation, Waltham, MA

Sandra Bailey, FHIMSS, Administrator, Methodist Hawyood Park Hospital, Brownsville, TN

Ron Contrado, FHIMSS, President, HOMISCO, Inc., Melrose, MA

Deborah Krau, FHIMSS Vice President, Information Services and CIO, Main Line Health System, Berwyn, PA

Gary Kurtz, FHIMSS, Administrative Director-IS, Geisinger Health System, Danville, PA

LaVone Neal, Director, Decision Support Services, Baylor Health Care System, Dallas, TX

Linda Reeder, RN, CHE, Sr. Clinical Applications Specialist, Intesys, Redmond, WA

Paul Vegoda, FHIMSS, Vice President and CIO, North Shore Health System, Great Neck, NY

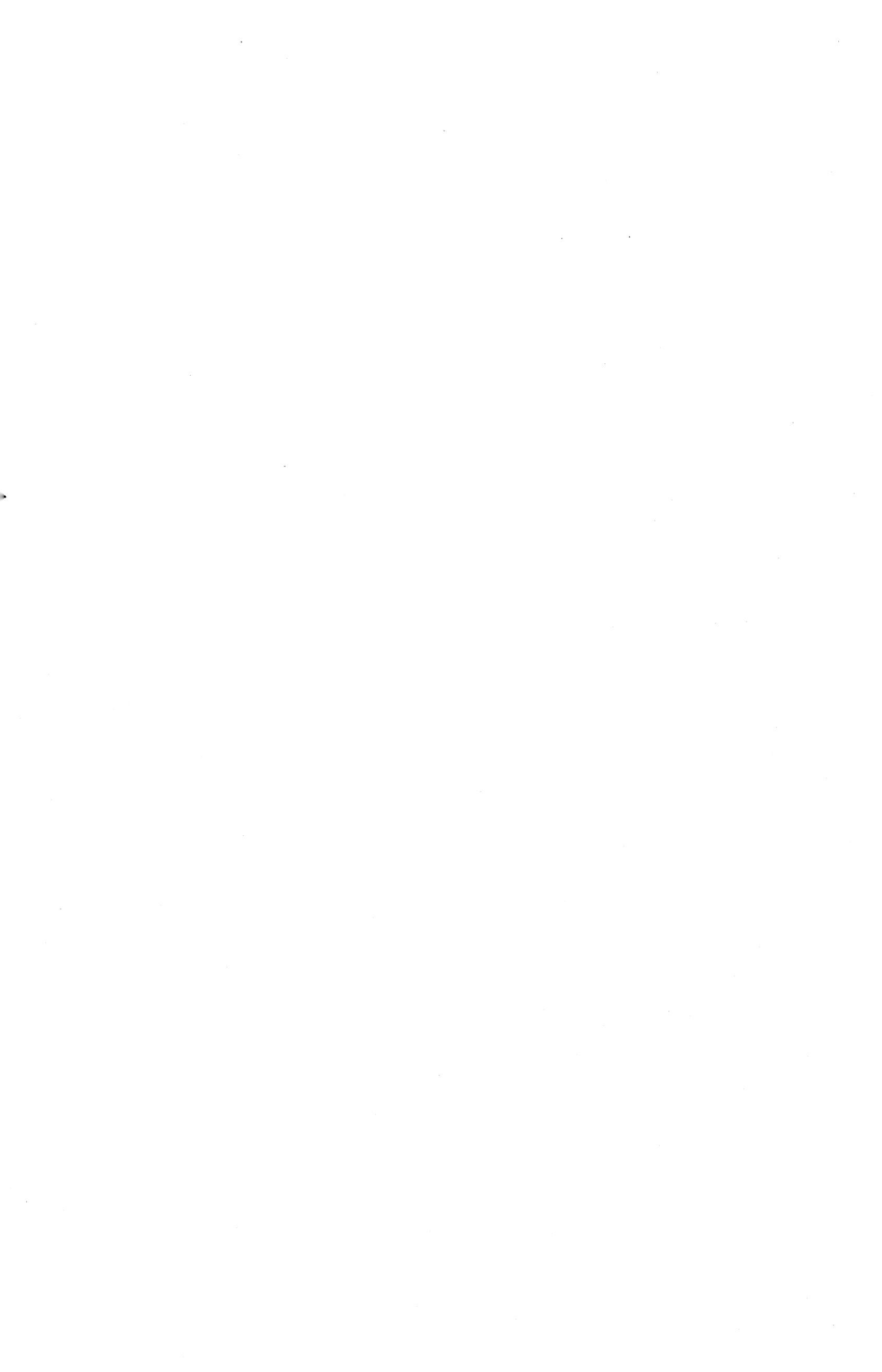

Healthcare Information and Management Systems Society Educational Events

HIMSS Long Term Care Information Systems Conference
August 31–September 2, 1998
New Orleans, LA

Telehealth Workshop
October 1–3, 1998
Dallas, TX

Introduction to Healthcare Information Management
October 21–23, 1998
Dallas, TX

Nursing Informatics
October 17, 1998
Salt Lake City, UT

Management Engineering Workshop
November 12–14, 1998
Atlanta, GA

All inquiries should be forwarded to:

Healthcare Information and Management Systems Society

mail: 230 East Ohio Street, Suite 600
Chicago, IL 60611–3201

phone: (312)664–HIMSS (4467)

fax: (312)664–6143

e-mail: himss@himss.org

web site: http://www.himss.org

fax back service: 800/HIMSS-11 (800/446–7711)

Ordering Information

HEALTHCARE INFORMATION MANAGEMENT®, published quarterly, is devoted to issues of significance in the professional development of individuals working in the areas of clinical systems, information systems, management engineering, and telecommunications.

SUBSCRIPTIONS cost $60.00 for individuals and $85.00 for institutions, agencies, and libraries. Standing orders are accepted. New York residents, add local sales tax. (For subscriptions outside the United States, orders must be prepaid in U.S. dollars by check drawn on a U.S. bank or charged to VISA, MasterCard, or American Express.)

SINGLE COPIES cost $22.00 plus shipping (see below) when payment accompanies order. California, New Jersey, New York, and Washington, D.C., residents please include appropriate sales tax. Canadian residents, add GST and any local taxes. Billed orders will be charged shipping and handling. No billed shipments to post office boxes. (Orders from outside the United States must be prepaid in U.S. dollars by check drawn on a U.S. bank or charged to VISA, MasterCard, or American Express.)

SHIPPING (Single Copies Only): $30.00 and under, add $5.50; to $50, add $6.50; to $75.00, add $7.50; to $100, add $9.00; to $150.00, add $10.00.

REPRINTS OF INDIVIDUAL ARTICLES: For quantities of 25 and under, contact the Healthcare Information and Management Systems Society, 230 East Ohio Street, Suite 600, Chicago, IL 60611-3201. Phone: (312) 664-4467. For quantities over 25, contact Vincent Fritzsche, Jossey-Bass Publishers, 350 Sansome Street, San Francisco, CA 94104-1342. Phone: (415) 433-1740, extension 3198.

MICROFILM copies of issues and articles are available in 16mm and 35mm, as well as microfiche in 105mm, through University Microfilms Inc., 300 North Zeeb Road, Ann Arbor, MI 48106-1346.

DISCOUNTS FOR QUANTITY ORDERS are available. Please write to the address below for information.

ALL ORDERS must include either the name of an individual or an official purchase order number. Please submit your orders as follows:

Subscriptions: specify issue (for example, HCIM 10:1) you would like subscription to begin with.

Single copies: specify volume and issue number.

MAIL orders to:
Jossey-Bass Publishers
350 Sansome Street
San Francisco, California 94104-1342

PHONE subscription or single-copy orders toll-free at (800) 956-7739 or at (415) 433-1767

FAX orders toll-free to: (800) 605-2665

LIBRARIANS are encouraged to contact the Periodicals Marketing Department at Jossey-Bass Publishers for a free sample issue.

VISIT THE JOSSEY-BASS HOME PAGE on the World Wide Web at www.josseybass.com for an order form or information about other titles of interest.